BIG PHARMA, WOMEN, AND T

In 2010, Thea Cacchioni testified before the US Food and Drug Administration against Flibanserin, a drug proposed to treat low sexual desire in women, dubbed the "pink Viagra" by the media. She was one of many academics and activists sounding the alarm about the lack of science behind the search for potentially lucrative sexual enhancement drugs for women.

In *Big Pharma, Women, and the Labour of Love*, Cacchioni moves beyond the search for a sexual pharmaceutical drug for women to ask a broader question: how does the medicalization of female sexuality already affect women's lives? Using in-depth interviews with doctors, patients, therapists, and other medical practitioners, Cacchioni shows that, whatever the future of the "pink Viagra," heterosexual women often now feel expected to take on the job of managing their and their partners' sexual desires. Their search for sexual pleasure can be a "labour of love," work that is enjoyable for some but a chore for others.

Original and insightful, Cacchioni's investigation will open up a wide-ranging discussion about the true impact of sexuality's medicalization.

THEA CACCHIONI is an assistant professor in the Department of Women's Studies at the University of Victoria.

THEA CACCHIONI

# Big Pharma, Women, and the Labour of Love

UNIVERSITY OF TORONTO PRESS
Toronto   Buffalo   London

© University of Toronto Press 2015
Toronto Buffalo London
www.utppublishing.com


ISBN 978-1-4426-4247-8 (cloth)
ISBN 978-1-4426-1137-5 (paper)

**Library and Archives Canada Cataloguing in Publication**

Cacchioni, Thea, 1976–, author
Big pharma, women, and the labour of love / Thea Cacchioni.

Includes bibliographical references and index. ISBN 978-1-4426-4247-8
(bound).—ISBN 978-1-4426-1137-5 (paperback)

1. Pharmaceutical industry—Social aspects.   2. Women—Sexual
behavior.   3. Women—Drug use.   4. Sexual disorders—Treatment.
I. Title.

HD9665.5.C32 2015      338.4'76151      C2015-902653-9

This book has been published with the help of a grant from the
Federation for the Humanities and Social Sciences, through the Awards
to Scholarly Publications Program, using funds provided by the Social
Sciences and Humanities Research Council of Canada.

University of Toronto Press acknowledges the financial assistance to its
publishing program of the Canada Council for the Arts and the Ontario
Arts Council, an agency of the Government of Ontario.

 **Canada Council Conseil des Arts**
**for the Arts du Canada**

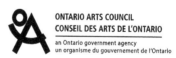 ONTARIO ARTS COUNCIL
CONSEIL DES ARTS DE L'ONTARIO
an Ontario government agency
un organisme du gouvernement de l'Ontario

University of Toronto Press acknowledges the financial support of the
Government of Canada through the Canada Book Fund for its publishing
activities.

# Contents

# Preface: Testifying at the US Food and Drug Administration

On 18 June 2010 I testified at a US Food and Drug Administration (FDA) advisory hearing on the drug Flibanserin, heralded by media as a "pink" Viagra for women. The day marked the culmination of my more than decade-long exploration of the pharmaceutical industry's attempts solve women's sexual problems with a drug following the blockbuster success of Viagra. Flibanserin, made by German pharmaceutical giant Boeringher Ingelheim (BI) is a serotonergic/adrenergic brain drug that BI claimed would be effective in the treatment of hypoactive sexual desire disorder (HSDD), a subset of female sexual dysfunction (FSD), the diagnosis increasingly used to define women's sexual problems in medical terms.

Before I took the stand, I marvelled at the collection of experts surrounding me. In front of me was Dr Irwin Goldstein, his wife Sue Goldstein, and Michelle King Robson, one of Goldstein's patients and founder and chair of EmpowHER, described as a "social health community" website for women. Dr Goldstein is one of the best-known, academically and commercially influential of the physicians who believe in the importance of finding a sexual enhancement drug for women. With ties to numerous pharmaceutical companies, he has been a spokesperson for Viagra since its release in 1999, and was hired by BI to endorse Flibanserin. Testimony on that side drew on the rhetoric of equality and "choice," based on the notion that, if men had their blue pill, women deserved a pink pill. The two women witnesses, both white and middle class, testified from the perspective of having been diagnosed (by Goldstein) with HSDD. They focused on their deep wish for a drug treatment for this "condition," which, they said, would help other women avoid the same consequences they had faced: diminished self-esteem and sense of womanhood, and in King Robson's case the end of her marriage. Unlike others who testified that day, King Robson did not declare whether or not she had any financial interest in the trial, but EmpowHER is a forum for drug company public relations, which, at the time of the trial, included BI-sponsored material on the woes of HSDD and the promise of Flibanserin.

Beside me were allies from the New View Campaign, ready to testify against the approval of Flibanserin. Chief among us was Leonore Tiefer, clinical psychologist, author, educator, and activist. Tiefer has dedicated her career to exposing the politics of the medicalization of sexuality and the rise of the sexual pharmaceutical industry. In 2000, she joined with other feminists to form the Working Group for a New View of Women's Sexual Problems, or New View. The mandate of the New View is to "challenge the distorted and oversimplified messages about sexuality that the pharmaceutical industry relies on to sell its new drugs" and "to expose biased research and promotional methods that serve corporate profit rather than people's pleasure and satisfaction" (http://www. newviewcampaign.org, para. 0). This was the second time representatives of the New View would testify against a sexual enhancement drug at an FDA hearing. The first was six years earlier, when they gathered to express concern over Proctor & Gamble's testosterone patch, Intrinsa. New View supporters have attended several key medical conferences organized by proponents of the FSD label since 2000, organized interdisciplinary counter-conferences, held press conferences, published books (Kaschak & Tiefer, 2001; Loe, 2004a), and special issues of journals (Cacchioni & Tiefer, 2012; Potts & Tiefer, 2006; Tiefer, 2008), formed a website (www.newviewcampaign.org), and a listserv. The New View has also created a classification system for understanding women's sexual complaints as an alternative to medical and pharmaceutical perspectives (see Chapter 1). This system acknowledges medical factors (many of which the New View argues are iatrogenic in nature), but positions sexual difficulties as shaped primarily by interrelated socio-cultural, political, economic, interpersonal, and psychological factors.

Although I too had critically examined the medicalization of women's sexual problems since the release of Viagra, I consider my collaboration with Tiefer and others on the Flibanserin trial to be my inaugural entry into the New View movement. In the days leading up to the FDA hearing, we met via Skype and then in person at our budget hotel a short drive from the Hilton where the advisory meeting was held. We created a series of "Fact Sheets" on topics such as "drugs and marketing" and "feminism and choice" to give to members of the press and

FDA panel members. We brought a petition with more than 763 signatures, gathered in just a few weeks. Fifteen experts on women's health and sexuality who could not attend the trial sent letters to the FDA supporting our perspective. Each of us did media interviews in our respective hometowns, and an interview with Tiefer was published on page one of the *New York Times* on the morning of the hearing (Wilson, 2010). Using her own funds, filmmaker Liz Canner, director of *Orgasm Inc: The Strange Science of Female Sexual Pleasure* (2011), rented a smaller room next door to the advisory hearing where her film played in a continuous loop. She hoped to offer the press and FDA panel members on their lunch breaks an alternative perspective to the multi-million-dollar public relations campaign BI had drummed up prior to the trial.

In support of the New View on women's sexual difficulties, we compiled twenty-seven peer-reviewed empirical studies on women's perceptions and experiences of sexual problems – we titled the studies "counter narratives" to BI's claims about the causes and effects of low sexual desire – and gave them to the advisory panel. Although the studies shed some light on socio-political factors that shape sexuality, like most research in this area they were predominantly quantitative, included the viewpoints of mainly heterosexual women, and were focused more on individual and interpersonal factors. Even so, they painted a more nuanced and complex picture of desire than BI's narrow view of desire as related strictly to neurological hardwiring.

As an example of the quantitative research we listed, DeLamater and Sill's (2005) survey of 1,348 men and women concludes that the main predictors of sexual desire are age, illness (excluding so-called HSDD), medication use, attitudes, expectations, quality of relationship, education, and household income. Hayes, Dennerstein, Bennet, Sidat, Gurrin, and Fairley's (2008) questionnaire of 1002 Australian women between the ages of twenty and seventy led them to the perhaps obvious conclusion that the duration of a sexual relationship is a primary determinant of the frequency of sexual desire. Carvalho and Nobre's (2010) mail-in questionnaire of 237 Portuguese women suggests a correlation between conservative sex beliefs and infrequent erotic thoughts. Dennerstein, Hayes, Sand, and Lehert's (2009) questionnaire of 1402 German and Italian women ages eighteen to sixty-five provides evidence that higher levels of interest in sex are associated with the quality of communication with one's partner and the tendency toward the sharing of daily activities. Koch, Mansfield, Thurau, and Carrey (2005) analyse data from a survey of 307 women's responses to a questionnaire about their sexual experiences; not surprisingly, they find that body image, sexual response, and sexual satisfaction are intimately linked. Another large-scale questionnaire, by Seal, Bradford, and Meston (2009) also links body esteem to frequency of sexual desire.

Of the few qualitative sources on our list, a semi-structured interview study of forty-four laywomen by Kleinplatz et al. (2009) demonstrates the ways in which "great sex" is associated with "connection, deep sexual and erotic intimacy, extraordinary communication, interpersonal risk-taking and exploration, authenticity, vulnerability, and transcendence" (p. 1). Nicholls' (2008) open-ended questionnaire of forty-nine women who defined themselves as having sexual difficulties concludes that women view their sexual problems as related far more to contextual factors than to individual psychological and medical factors.

On the day of the hearing, our own testimonies focused more specifically on problems related to Flibanserin's safety, side effects, efficacy, clinical trials methodology, and marketing. The pill was tested in phase-3 trials[1] on 5,000 pre-menopausal women diagnosed with HSDD in North America and Europe. All the women were in heterosexual, monogamous relationships of one year or longer, with an average length of eleven years. In its public statements, BI focused only on data from North American studies, which included only 1,300 women. The clinical trial participants were asked to evaluate their sexual desire and activities, recording "sexually satisfying events" (SSEs), a subjective measure determined by the woman participating in the clinical trial.[2] The use of SSEs as an endpoint is an industry standard for judging the success of sexual pharmaceutical drugs proposed to treat FSD. Researchers found that women who took Flibanserin had only an extra 0.7 of an SSE per month compared with the group taking a placebo – not a large degree of success considering the potential risks associated with taking a daily drug whose long-term effects were unknown. Indeed, 14 per cent of the participants withdrew from Flibanserin's clinical trials due to side effects such as "dizziness, nausea, fatigue, somnolence, and insomnia" (United States, 2010, p. 117).

In my testimony, I focused on the marketing of Flibanserin and the disorder the drug was meant to treat. In the lead-up to the trial, BI had hired the world-renowned public relations firm GFK Healthcare to produce a website called "Sex, Brain, Body." Billed as an "educational campaign," the website's aim was to convince visitors that one in ten women suffers from HSDD, "a persistent or recurrent decrease or lack of sexual desire" (Cacchioni, 2010, p. 2) As I testified, this "thinly veiled marketing campaign, complete with celebrity endorsement" used several different mechanisms to suggest that HSDD is a valid neurological condition affecting one in ten women, despite the complete absence of peer-reviewed research to support the claim. I explained that there was no research to support the notion that there is an empirical, baseline level of "normal" desire or that norms of desire vary from era to era and culture to culture. I also argued that desire is not an internal, physiological drive, but rather is shaped by numerous interpersonal and socio-political determinants. Drawing on the New View classification system for women's sexual problems, I noted that quality of sex education, poor body images, experiences of sexual violence or trauma, relationship problems, sexism, shame over sexual fantasies, stress, and length of relationship all shape our "level" of desire. I concluded by pointing out that even the highly medicalized American Psychiatric Association had decided to remove HSDD from the upcoming fifth edition of the *Diagnostic and Statistical Manual of Mental Disorders* (American Psychiatric Association, 2013). Since the FDA panel members were aware that they could not approve a drug without a valid diagnosis for it to treat, this point caused some confused looks and even some paper shuffling, as BI had carefully avoided this update when presenting its data. Flibanserin was denied approval that day, but the comments of FDA panellists suggested that they took poor efficacy and safety concerns more seriously than our critique of the HSDD nomenclature.

When I returned to my home city of Vancouver, British Columbia, I awaited news about the fate of Flibanserin in the Canadian context. In any event, I would not have the chance to testify at a Canadian counterpart to the FDA hearing: under the Canadian system, drug companies can meet with regulatory authorities while their drug is under review, and they often bring in their own paid, academic experts, but there is no chance for an independent expert witness to counter their claims. I suspected that BI would drop its case in other countries, including Canada, if it could not capture the profitable US market, and so it did.

The Flibanserin trial is just one page in the book of the brave new world of sex drugs in the sexual pharmaceutical era. Following the financial success of Viagra and other erectile enhancement drugs, Big Pharma has dedicated millions of dollars to the search for a sexual enhancement drug for women. Viagra has not been a panacea for the vast majority of men's sexual problems, and its risks have turned out to be much greater than makers Pfizer Inc. would have us believe (including loss of eyesight and increased rate of heart attacks) (Edwards, 2010; Mitka, 2000). Yet the drug industry has gone to great lengths to cash in on the estimated US$1.7 billion dollar market for sex drugs for women (Hartley, 2006). The pursuit of a "pink" Viagra has led to a variety of efforts to construct "female sexual dysfunction" as a diagnostic label with international medical legitimacy. Some industry hopefuls and social commentators have lauded these developments as evidence of a "second sexual revolution" (Hutton, 2003, 0), with science, medicine, and Big Pharma hard at work to guarantee women's sexual pleasure.

As reflected most clearly in the work of the New View Campaign, all this has raised major concerns on the part of feminist scholars, activists, and health practitioners, who are highlighting the health and social risks of the pharmaceutical industry's growing influence over definitions of health and illness, the socio-political and interpersonal roots of the vast majority of women's sexual dissatisfactions, and the limitations of narrowly drawn norms guiding how "sex" – especially, "good sex" – is defined (Kaschak & Tiefer, 2001)

# Acknowledgments

This book has been my own labour of love, with many supporters along the way. First and foremost, I would like to thank the women who participated in my research, who have my deepest gratitude for their honesty and reflection.

My work and career path have been shaped by two key mentors: Carol Wolkowitz, who went above and beyond for me as my MA and PhD supervisor and helped me theorize the labour of love; and Leonore Tiefer, founder of the New View Campaign. Leonore taught me so much of what I know about the sexual pharmaceutical industry and encouraged me to translate my academic work into activism. The work and activism of sexual medicine critics such as Virginia Braun, Liz Canner, Nicola Gavey, Carol Groneman, Kristina Gupta, Karen Hicks, Amber Hui, Meika Loe, Rachel Leibert, Barbara Marshall, Annie Potts, Judy Segal, and Jennifer Terry have also been influential.

I am indebted to the Ruth Wynn Woodward endowment and the Department of Gender, Sexuality, and Women's Studies at Simon Fraser University for supporting me in organizing the "Medicalization of Sex" conference in 2010, an event that had a major influence on my thinking in this field. I would also like to thank all of the students who have taken my "Medicalization of Sex" class over the years. Your engagement has pushed my critical thinking.

I've had the pleasure of teaching and researching at the University of Warwick in the United Kingdom, the University of British Columbia (UBC) Okanagan, UBC Vancouver, Simon Fraser University, and, more recently, my home department in Gender Studies at the University of Victoria. Numerous faculty and staff in each of these institutions offered valuable support along the way.

This book evolved over time with feedback from many. Thank you to Douglas Hildebrand at the University of Toronto Press for your ongoing guidance in this endeavour and for selecting three excellent anonymous peer reviewers for this book; I am eternally grateful for their insightful feedback on previous drafts. Thank you to my research assistant Erin Fuller for your careful referencing work and to Kyla Slobodin for your help theorizing, proof reading, and completing the bibliography. Thank you to Barry Norris for your thorough copy-editing work.

An extra thanks to the journals that have given me permission to reprint revised sections of previously published material. Parts of Cacchioni & Wolkowitz (2011) and Farrell & Cacchioni (2012) appear in Chapter 2; much of Cacchioni (2007) is featured in Chapters 5 and 6. I thank co-authors Janine Farrell and Carol Wolkowitz for their permission.

Last but not least, thank you to my family – my mom, especially – friends, and my love, for all your encouragement and distraction along the way.

# BIG PHARMA, WOMEN, AND THE LABOUR OF LOVE

# Introduction: The Labour of Love in the Sexual Pharmaceutical Era

As the significant critique of the medicalization of women's sexual problems in the sexual pharmaceutical era unfolded in academic, media, and activist circles, I could not help but notice how infrequently we heard from women who identify as having sexual problems. In the vast polemic that formed between expert proponents and critics of sexual pharmaceuticals, there was little analysis of how women who define themselves as having sexual problems understand these issues; what strategies, if any, they draw on to address them in everyday life; and how low-tech, high-tech, medicalized, non-medicalized, and demedicalized strategies compare. Angel (2012) notes that the near-exclusive focus on sexual pharmaceuticals in the existing critique "glosses over resources such as women's magazines and self-help books, for instance, which speak in an emotional, psychological, *and* behavioural register" (p. 12). In keeping with the aim of this book, she suggests that we "widen the lens of criticism" to include the regulatory and disciplinary aspects of sexual improvement as found in self-help, even seemingly feminist material. I similarly contend that an analysis of some of the everyday strategies for understanding and solving women's sexual problems will provide a more nuanced look at the politics of the sexual pharmaceutical industry and overall work of (hetero) sexual improvement.

My hope is that this book will reach the various audiences that might seem – or, in fact, are – at odds with one another: biomedical experts, feminist sociologists and sexologists, and women who perceive themselves as having sexual problems. The politics of how drug companies, scientists, and doctors have approached the development of a sexual pharmaceutical drug for women has been thoroughly critiqued (see, for example, Moynihan & Mintzes, 2010). However, I explore a different, but entirely related, set of questions: How do women perceive their sexual problems? What do they do to address them? What factors influence their perceptions and choices? What do these strategies (from pharmaceutical to self-help) have in common? How do they differ? What do they tell us about medicalization? What do they tell us about (hetero) sexual norms?

I argue that, despite sophisticated efforts, drug companies and sexual medicine physicians so far have failed in their vision to create a market of pill-popping women diagnosed with female sexual dysfunction (FSD). Two drugs hyped by industry and media have been denied approval by the US Food and Drug Administration (FDA), and the search for the "pink" Viagra is now frequently cited as a case study of "disease mongering" and Big Pharma corruption (Moynihan & Mintzes, 2010). This is no surprise. As my research has found, many women perceive the socio-political and interpersonal context of their sexual experiences as the primary determinant shaping their sexual dissatisfaction, and are aware that their sexual responses, feelings, and abilities are judged in relation to narrowly defined notions of "normal" sexual functioning. Yet despite recognizing normative sexual ideals as a constraint, many women *work* to achieve this sexual script, rather than challenge it.

The most socially celebrated and medically validated sexual script is frequent sexual desire, high arousal, and orgasm as endpoint, ideally in the context of heterosexual monogamy. In the context of heterosex, the key ingredient is penis-vagina intercourse, with all other sexual activities relegated to "foreplay," not "real" sex. Just as hegemonic constructions linking erection with successful masculinity influence men's perceptions of their erectile difficulties (Loe, 2001), women in my study who experienced chronic genital pain leading to disinterest in or refusal to engage in sexual intercourse felt the most ostracized from sexual norms. Sexual pain represents one of the four subsets of FSD, and yet feminist critics have said little about the politics of its medicalization.

Thus, whether or not a safe and effective sexual enhancement drug for women ever materializes, and whether or not a woman is diagnosed with FSD, it seems that women who do not conform to idealized sexual standards feel they are expected to spend time and effort on "the labour of love" (Cacchioni, 2007). In the context of this discussion, the labour of love refers to the unacknowledged effort and the continuing monitoring that women are expected to devote to managing their and their partner's sexual desires and activities. In this sense, it can be seen as a kind of "sex work." Pressures on women to learn to perform specific sexual behaviours are especially naturalized through the sexual and emotional division of labour in heterosexual relationships (Duncombe & Marsden, 1996). Some women, depending on various factors, might perceive sex work as "empowering" (Cacchioni & Wolkowitz, 2011); for others, it is a "chore" (Cacchioni, 2007). Although it can be enjoyable to approach sex work as a way of honing one's sexual "talents" (Tiefer, 1995), women have been called on disproportionately – indeed, compelled – to do so since the twentieth-century liberalization, commodification, and (re)medicalization of sex. As I argue, sexual "functioning" is now part and parcel of women's sexual capital.

There are, of course, alternatives to the sex work imperative. One form of refusing sex work is what one might term "queering" the heteronormative script against which sexual "function" and "dysfunction" typically are judged. Queering in this context can be understood as undoing the normative script, accepting what feels good over achieving, performing, or avoiding sexual norms – a path that can be taken in or outside the context of heterosexuality. Queering sex, however, is only one way to resist sex work. In my study, none of the women in this study explicitly identified as "asexual," as a growing number of individuals in the West have self-proclaimed (Fahs, 2010; Scherrer, 2008), but some were positive about forgoing sexual relationships in favour of prioritizing non-sexual activities, relationships, and lifestyles. I argue that queering (hetero) sex and/or embracing asexuality or non-sexuality represents a challenge to hegemonic practices. Yet many women who adopt these strategies face social, interpersonal, and economic consequences. Therefore, I also argue that challenging heterosexual norms at the level of sexual practices does not entirely destabilize or crumble the institution of heterosexuality.

### Researching the Labour of Love in the Sexual Pharmaceutical Era

In researching this book, I drew on what Judith Jack Halberstam (1994) terms a "scavenger" methodology. I examined the labour of love in the sexual pharmaceutical era by drawing on (a) portrayals of women's sexual problems as bodily problems best treated by a drug, found in, for example, academic journal articles, medical texts, industry-sponsored conferences, drug company press releases, magazine articles, advertisements, websites, best-selling books, and television and radio appearances; (b) interdisciplinary academic and activist critiques of the medicalization of women's sexual problems, as expressed in academic journal articles, books, conferences and "counter-conferences," FDA hearings, blogs, emails, and listservs; and (c) my own qualitative, empirical research into lay and expert perceptions of women's sexual difficulties and strategies for dealing with them. For the purposes of this study, I did not interview any men about their experiences of their own or their partner's sexual difficulties, although I believe this would be a valuable direction for future research.

Although quantitative methods are important for feminist research (Oakley, 2005), like others who have researched similar themes – for instance, Duncombe & Marsden (1996); Gavey (1993, 2005); Holland, Romazanoglu, Sharpe, & Thomson (1998); Kaler (2006); Nicolson & Burr (2003); Potts (2002); Thompson (1990, 1995)– I chose qualitative research as a way to gather "rich," in-depth data. The style of qualitative research I conducted was informed by my feminist and social justice principles, "emphasizing non-exploitative, non-hierarchical approaches to research subjects" (O'Connell Davidson & Layder, 1994, p. 50), and a critical examination of "how we know what we know" about the information we collect (Holland et al., 1998, p. 459). In other words, throughout my research, I made every effort to ensure informed consent and confidentiality, and to make interview participants comfortable at every stage. I also attempted to reflect on the biases I might have brought to the project design and analysis.

The research was conducted in my home city of Vancouver, but there were several other reasons for choosing this location for my fieldwork. As a site of research, Vancouver allowed me to interview women from a wide range of social locations. Although it is an expensive and increasingly unaffordable city, Vancouver is nonetheless diverse in relation to social class, race, ethnicity, religion, and sexuality. In addition, as in an increasing number of urban locales in North America and Europe, Vancouver's main hospital has a sexual medicine unit. This unit deals with sexual paraphelia and sexual dysfunctions and is covered by provincial health insurance with a referral by a general practitioner (GP). I was fortunate to know somebody with a personal connection to a doctor in this unit, thus enabling my research access.

Not wanting my research to reflect solely the viewpoints of women with the will and social capital to seek medical advice for their sexual difficulties, I also advertised the study throughout the city on bulletin boards in coffee shops, community centres, and sex toy stores, and on the streets of low- and high-income neighbourhoods. I eventually found advertising in a free local community newspaper to be the most effective recruitment strategy for the community sample. The advertisement I placed in the sexual medicine clinic and throughout the community was extremely simple. It was printed on university letterhead in a twelve-point font and called for the voluntary participation of women over the age of nineteen who identified as having any kind of sexual difficulty. I did not offer a financial incentive, just a chance to reflect on one's sexual difficulties. Like the consent form, the long version of the ad explained the details of the study protocol. Participants filled out a brief questionnaire about their age, partnership, education, profession, number of children under their care, first language, country of origin, and self-described race, class, ethnicity, and religion. Interviews were semi-structured, lasting approximately one hour, either in my home or at a place of the participant's convenience, and participants could opt out of the interview at any time. I explained that the names and identify-revealing information of participants would be changed, transcripts safely stored for twenty-five years, and interviews themed and coded manually.

Although I consider myself a deeply ethical researcher, one of the greatest challenges in this process was negotiating the medical gatekeeping that surrounded my access to patients in the sexual medicine unit. I was struck by the comparative ease with which medical students wanting to learn more about sexual medicine were able to observe patient-doctor interactions and even examine patients. I had been trained extensively in ethical interviewing, yet the physicians were adamant that I not be allowed to observe doctor-patient clinical sessions. Instead, they would allow me only to advertise the interview portion of my study to their patients via signs in the waiting room and a direct mail-out completed by their administrative staff. Even after I had obtained hospital ethics approval, doctors at the sexual medicine unit deemed that surveillance of me was necessary. Therefore, they asked me to participate in mock pilot interviews with two sexual medicine nurses while a physician observed me through a two-way mirror. Luckily, I passed the test, with just a few suggestions on how to word questions about sexual experiences – for example, beginning a question with the phrase, "If I may ask."

Throughout the process, I came to understand the paradoxical nature of designing, conducting, and analysing social research on a sensitive matter. It was challenging to find women willing to talk about their sexual problems and practitioners willing to talk about their work, as it was increasingly embroiled in controversy. I spent months preparing the research design and then waiting for participants to trickle in. I tried to gauge the extent of the medicalization of women's sexual problems without contributing to unnecessary medicalization via the "labeling effect" (Kimmel, 1988, p. 81). I asked women to divulge highly personal information about themselves without replicating a Foucaultian-style "confessional" (Foucault, 1979). I attempted to avoid positioning myself as an expert or a counsellor on women's sexual problems, but could not help but console women as they told me about their past experiences of depression, mental, physical, and sexual abuse, and relationship turmoil.

After a solid year of advertising my study, I managed to conduct semi-structured, in-depth, qualitative interviews with thirty-one women (see the Appendix). To avoid the empirical exercise of the researcher labelling and defining the research participants, the questionnaire I crafted to gather information about their identities was open-ended, allowing them to self-identify various aspects of their identities, albeit with the assumption that they would define themselves as "women over the age of 19," as stipulated in the advertisement. Twenty-seven participants identified as heterosexual, one as lesbian, and three as bisexual. The women ranged in age from twenty-one to sixty-two (the average age was thirty-three), and identified with seven different ethnicities and eight different nationalities. Of significance, the majority who appeared to be of northern European decent described themselves straightforwardly as "white Canadian," whereas, reflecting their racialization in the Canadian context, women from all other racial and ethnic backgrounds marked themselves in more specific terms – for example, "Indo-Canadian," "Italian-Canadian," "Japanese-Canadian," "Chinese-Canadian," or "Eurasian." Only two indigenous women were in the study, one self-identified as xʷməθkʷəy̓əm (Musqueam) and one as Māori. Ultimately, the sample was fairly diverse in terms of self-described ethnicity, nationality, occupation, social class, type of sexual problems, and strategies for dealing with them, but predominantly white, middle class, gender conforming, and heterosexual, much like the target audience so far for sexual pharmaceutical drugs.

Although the majority described themselves as middle class, one woman lived below the poverty line and one-third described themselves as working class. Their education ranged from two who had not completed high school to two who had a PhD. Their occupations included gas station attendant, sex worker, student, waiter, documentary film maker, actor, hospital attendant, school teacher, yoga teacher, stay-at-home mother, lab technician, and scientist, among others. These women identified as having a range of often-overlapping sexual difficulties with desire, arousal, orgasm, and pain, and had sought the services of GPs, sexual medicine physicians, pelvic physiotherapists, homeopaths, naturopaths, energy healers, psychiatrists, psychologists, counsellors, sex therapists, and self-help sources. Eleven had experienced some form of sexual pain, mainly as a result of chronic genital pain. This was an unexpected feature of the research, and sparked my further investigation into the complexity of biomedical, psychological, and sociological/ social constructionist understandings of chronic genital pain (Cacchioni & Wolkowitz, 2011; Farrell & Cacchioni, 2012).

Interviews usually took place at my apartment, because it offered privacy. At the beginning of the interview, I offered participants tea and made a bit of "small talk" to put us both at ease. On the advice of sexual health clinicians at the sexual medicine unit, I made tissues available. Although many interviews were somewhat lighthearted, these tissues came in handy when some women spoke about issues relating to depression and negative relationship experiences such as mental, physical, and sexual violence. In particular, interviewees who had not previously sought expert advice for their sexual difficulties expressed gratitude for having a chance to discuss these issues with a stranger. Similar to Loe's (2004a) experience when she talked to men about their "Viagra stories," several women claimed I was the first person they had ever talked to about these issues in any depth.

I also undertook in-depth, semi-structured interviews with five practitioners who treat women's sexual difficulties, including one sex therapist, two pelvic physiotherapists, and one sexual medicine specialist from a local hospital's sexual medicine unit, all white women in their forties. I eventually was granted access to observe several sexual medicine "rounds" over a year, where doctors (typically three women and three men, all white) discussed their cases and appropriate treatments, developed protocols, and had informal discussions. I observed pelvic physiotherapy sessions over the span of two afternoons wherein one pelvic physiotherapist asked her clients if they would allow a sociologist to observe the session. The four women observed were white and in their twenties or thirties, and had occupations ranging from secretary to university professor. The physiotherapist explained to them that

I would not reveal their identity and that they could ask me to leave at any time. Understanding the vulnerability women might feel during this intimate procedure, I sat behind the client's shoulders during the examination and other procedures involving nudity, and recorded my observations after, rather than during, each session; see Cacchioni & Wolkowitz (2011) for more discussion of these sessions. Finally, I attended a range of sex-related community events, including workshops for women with sexual pain.

As O'Connell Davidson and Layder (1994) remark, feminist researchers believe in the value of "continually reflecting upon the ways in which their own social identity and values affect the data they are gathering and the picture of social reality they are producing" (p. 52). While conducting this research, I noted several important factors affecting the interview process. My gender might have given me insider status with the women I interviewed, and might have helped make them feel more comfortable during the interview process. In one particular interview, however, a Chinese-Canadian woman in her fifties did not open up to me to the extent that others did. There could be several reasons for this, but my being a white, middle-class researcher in her late twenties – and thus our differences in race, class, and age – might have influenced the extent of her comfort level and trust.

When analysing the research data, I attempted to strike a balance between noticing what seemed to be fairly hegemonic constructions, beliefs, ideals, or practices within an urban North American locale such as Vancouver, and perhaps even more generally "Western" capitalist societies, and recognizing how intersecting aspects of identity might influence the ways in which one constructs, engages with, accepts, rejects, or is included or excluded by these paradigms. As my research was decidedly inductive, my theoretical framework was informed by grounded theory (Glaser, 2002), which allows research findings to shape the theoretical framework. Unlike positivist writings, which start with a hypothesis and an attending theory, I wanted the data to guide my empirical and theoretical findings and conclusions.

## Contextualizing the Labour of Love in the Sexual Pharmaceutical Era

Two interrelated processes form the basis of the labour of love in the sexual pharmaceutical era: the rise of (bio)medicalization and the social construction of heteronormativity in narrow terms. Although both social processes have been thoroughly challenged and resisted, they remain firmly entrenched in many ways. One might question the value of researching a category as privileged as normative heterosex, but I approach this identity, institution, and set of practices in a similar way that critical race theorists have approached "whiteness" (Frankenberg, 1993). I am interested in unpacking an essentialized, taken-for-granted, and celebrated social category, and highlighting how it is naturalized through numerous processes and even, as we will see, "hard work."

### (Bio)medicalization

The Viagra era reflects a *medicalized* understanding of men's and women's sexual identities, practices, and bodily experiences. The concept of medicalization emerged in the 1960s to explain the increasing power of medical concepts, institutions, and individual figures of authority, following the professionalization and expansion of medicine in the late nineteenth century (Conrad, 1992). It typically refers to the process wherein "more and more areas of everyday life have come under medical dominion, influence, and supervision" (Zola, 1983, p. 295). Over the years, a range of behaviours and practices once seen as "good," "bad," or just "normal" – for example, homosexuality (until it was demedicalized in the official literature in 1973), depression, social anxiety, and addiction to drinking and gambling – came to be understood within the lexicon of health and illness. The proliferation of medicalization has led to the development of what Rose and Novas (2005) refer to as "biological citizenship" – the identification of citizenship as based on vital characteristics. According to Foucault (1979), the subtle but powerful disciplinary technology of "biopower" – the administration of bodies and the calculated management of life – is a mode of governmentality unique to modern nation-states. Although Foucault did not focus on its use in colonization, biopower is, as Morgensen (2011) argues, a powerful colonial mechanism.

The medicalization of sex can be traced to the late nineteenth century, when Western science, medicine, and the emergent field of sexology generally superseded custom and religion as authorities on sex. As Digby (1989) contends, the Age of Enlightenment "validated the role of the professional" and "virtually extinguished the female healers" (p. 195). Gynecology offered "lucrative opportunities" if the practice was to expand to affluent women. Psychiatry, another relatively new area of medical specialization, was inextricably linked with gynecology in its attempt to "solve" sexual variation and deviance. As seen in the rise of diagnoses such as nymphomania, hysteria, frigidity, and inversion, some women were constructed as "in need of management" and potentially sexually dangerous. In this medical climate, "even minor transgressions of the social strictures that defined 'feminine' could be classified as diseased" (Groneman, 1994, p. 341). Again, the timing of this strict regulation of white femininity in the nineteenth century was no coincidence. The violence integral to colonization and nation building were justified by falsely constructing white bodies as especially predisposed to rationality and sexual restraint (Fausto-Sterling, 1995).

As Leonore Tiefer and I have argued elsewhere (Cacchioni & Tiefer, 2012), Western scientific and medical views on sexual norms and deviance have changed over time. While, in the nineteenth century, sexual deviance was seen as largely the result of biological shortcomings, by the turn of the century Freud's psychoanalytic perspective of sexuality had gained popularity. Moving away from the Enlightenment tendency towards biological determinism, Freud emphasized psychosexual development as the leading factor in shaping sexual behaviour, identity, and practice. Eventually Kinsey's mid-twentieth-century large-scale surveys of sexual behaviour in the United States gave rise to a behaviouralist model of sex, highlighting and even celebrating sexual variation. A humanistic approach to understanding and exploring sex followed as part of the "sexual revolution" of the 1970s. Humanistic sexology distanced itself from biological reductionism and physical norms, and prided itself on creative, mind-body approaches to tapping into sexual pleasure (Tiefer, 2006a).

Contemporary sexology is now divided between or reflects a mixture of biological determinism, psychoanalysis, behaviouralism, and humanism, but the biological branch of sexology has garnered the most legitimacy and funding in the academic research community (Tiefer, 2001, 2008, 2012). Masters and Johnson's work from the 1960s onwards marked a return to an emphasis on the physiological workings of sex through their universal human sexual response cycle (HSRC), derived from laboratory studies of "human sex." The HSRC, formed on the basis of a small, homogeneous sample of individuals who were told what outcomes would be seen as "successful" (Tiefer, 2001), links sexual functioning to the performance of a supposedly normal "sequence of genital functions" (Tiefer, 2006a, p. 283). This model of universal sexual functioning has been the basis of the sexual "dysfunction" nomenclature in the American Psychiatric Association's *Diagnostic and Statistical*

*Manual of Mental Disorders* since the 1980s. But despite their emphasis on the measurement of genital response using high-tech devices, until the invention of sexual pharmaceuticals Masters and Johnson and other big names in sexology mainly recommended psychosexual education and behavioural therapy to improve sexual satisfaction. As Tiefer (2008) argues, once the drug industry took an interest in funding research to support this model, the "marginalized field of psychosocial sexology abandoned its humanistic heritage and capitulated to the dominant medical model" (p. 453).

Scholars critically examining the sexual pharmaceutical era have not only added to the canon of classic medicalization scholarship; they have also been influenced by and influenced new theories on what is termed "biomedicalization" (Clarke, Mamo, Fishman, Shim, & Fosket, 2003, p. 162), or what Conrad has more conservatively dubbed "the shifting engines of medicalization" (Conrad, 2007, p. 14; Conrad & Leiter, 2004).[1] Whereas medicalization was once the province mainly of doctors and hospitals, a complex web that includes drug companies, advertising agencies, public relations firms, health maintenance organizations (in the United States), and insurance companies currently bolsters this social process. Critics who draw on biomedicalization theory argue that drug companies now have an unparalleled influence over understandings of health and illness through the funding of medical research, conferences, and continuing medical education, and by hiring medical spokespeople and public relations, marketing, and advertising firms for the direct-to-consumer advertising of both drugs and the conditions they claim to treat (see, for example, Fishman & Mamo 2001; Katz & Marshall, 2003; Loe, 2004a; Tiefer, 2001). Women are under ever-increasing pressure in this biomedical era to use the HPV vaccination, pharmaceutical means of birth control, and hormone replacement therapy (Rochon Ford & Saibil, 2009).

Fuelled by the blockbuster success of Viagra and other sexual pharmaceuticals, the field of sexual medicine is surely a product of biomedicalization. As Tiefer (2006b) has outlined, urologists in the 1980s initially brought men's erections into their domain as a way of expanding their limited and dwindling repertoire of expertise and client base. In an attempt to legitimize erectile problems as a serious medical concern, they focused on the physiological aspects of erections, downplaying psycho-social solutions in favour of promoting penile injections or permanent penile implants. It was not until the introduction of Viagra that urologists were able to offer a more attractive solution to men's erectile difficulties and gain the legitimacy they have in the wider profession today. When Viagra was released, hospital urology departments blossomed into interdisciplinary sexual medicine units. In a very short period, clinicians and researchers working on sexual dysfunction were the beneficiaries of generous industry funding. Of this funding, Sandra Leiblum, a sex therapist who has worked in several different sexual medicine centres once commented, "we need the money. The field would be stagnant without it. Otherwise we'd be sitting around drinking tea at some university" (quoted in Loe, 2004a, p. 134). Leiblum's wish to do more than "drink tea at some university" suggests that the perceived marginal status of sexual medicine might have inspired renewed efforts to (re)medicalize women's sexual problems.

Indeed, although claiming to adopt a "biopsychosocial" approach (Krychman & Kingsberg, 2013, p. 113), sexual medicine clearly emphasizes the bio, then the psycho, and rarely the social theorizations of sex and the body. As Julia Heiman, director of the Kinsey Institute, once claimed, "[p]sycho-social analyses [of sexual problems] can be done but they aren't usually because they don't communicate anything to one's colleagues and there's no reimbursement for that. It's really a guild issue" (quoted in Loe, 2004a, p. 34). Since sexual medicine might have to prove its legitimacy in ways that other medical sub-specialties do not, quotes such as these suggest that sexual medicine specialists fear that "psycho-social" analyses might jeopardize the legitimacy the field has managed to gain.

Biomedicalization is part and parcel of a greater shift towards a neoliberal conceptualization of the self, with an emphasis on individualism, self-discipline, efficiency, and commodified social relations. Maximizing one's health has become a mandatory requirement of the self, causing some scholars to challenge the morality of "healthism" (Crawford, 1980), or even writing "against health" (Metzl & Kirkland, 2010). Critics of the neoliberal imperative argue that the assumption of individual control over the fate of one's health ignores social, economic, political, and environmental factors that shape health inequalities. This framework also suggests that we can meet hegemonic standards through the purchase of goods and services (Cruikshank, 1999). As Rose (2007) argues, "biology is no longer destiny," but "our somatic, corporeal, neurochemical individuality now becomes a field of choice, prudence, and responsibility" (p. 40). This individualized and commodified framework is evident in recent breast cancer awareness campaigns (King, 2006, 2010), self-esteem workshops for empowering people living in poverty (Cruikshank, 1999), and sex, relationship, career, and health advice geared towards women's liberal equality, as seen in a variety of media (Becker, 2004; Hawkes, 1996).

In line with neoliberal governmentality, "sexuality is talked about in the idiom of health promotion and lifestyle choices" (Jackson & Scott, 1997, p. 557). On the one hand, a healthy lifestyle is seen as preventing sexual decline; as Katz and Marshall (2003) point out, the medical literature is rife with suggestions for "eating a low fat diet, performing cardiovascular exercise, reducing alcohol consumption, and refraining from smoking" (p.11) as preventative measures to age-related sexual decline. But a new *sex as health* message (Gupta, 2011; Marshall, 2012) has also emerged in the medical and self-help literature that frames sex as a *health-giving* activity, particularly for those approaching their senior years. As Kristina Gupta and I have discussed (Gupta & Cacchioni, 2013), the sex-as-health imperative might be even more pervasive than the medicalization of women's sexual problems via the pharmaceutical industry's efforts towards the discovery and marketing of a "pink" Viagra.

The impetus towards sexual improvement is also guided by "post-feminist" ideologies, a kind of "sexualism" that at times promotes highly commodified, goal-oriented, and even medicalized frameworks for understanding women's sexual pleasure, the importance of it, and how to realize it (McCaughey & French, 2001). Despite the promise of sexual liberation as propounded by feminist sex manuals and toy shops, sexual improvement self-help arguably falls under the category of "life politics" – transformation focused on the individual's body, rather than on structural change or collective emancipation (Giddens, 1991). Critics such as Ebert (1996) question whether body-pleasure projects can ever radicalize or destabilize what McCaughey and French (2001) term "an individualistic, capitalist consumption model" of sexual improvement and pleasure, since "these projects fail to criticize the commodification inherent in them" (p. 91).

Finally, critical discussions of the sexual pharmaceutical era thus far have focused on the growing power of medicine, but medicalization theorists have always allowed for a discussion of the limits of medical power. As early as 1979, Phil Strong pointed to various institutional constraints prohibiting doctors from exercising more power. He highlighted the role of the state in "limiting medical expansion" and safeguarding "bourgeois freedom," as well as the role of the "questioning" and "litigious" lay public in limiting medical expansion (Strong, 1979,

p. 210, quoted in Williams, 2001, p. 139). More recently, Light (2000) has argued that physicians face a number of "countervailing powers" through a series of institutional constraints, while Conrad and Leiter (2004) further demonstrate how insurance companies might prohibit increased medicalization. Similarly, Foucault viewed doctors' role in medicalization as "links in a set of power relations," rather than as "figures of domination" (1984, p. 247; see also Jones & Porter, 1997; Petersen & Bunton, 2000). Over thirty years ago, feminist critic Catherine Riessman (1983) argued that medicalization was a "contradictory reality" for women, "part of the problem and the solution" (p. 59), a process whereby "women have both gained and lost with each (medical) intrusion" (p. 47).

*Heteronormativity*

A *heteronormative* understanding of men's and women's sexual identities, practices, and bodily experiences is also at the heart of the sexual pharmaceutical era's medicalized approach to sex. Heteronormativity refers specifically to "the normative status of heterosexuality which renders any alternative sexualities 'other' and marginal" (Jackson, 1999, p. 16; see also Richardson, 1996). As Tiefer (1995) famously once wrote, "sex is not a natural act," but is produced by the social world. Jackson (1999) cites three mutually reinforcing levels of heteronormativity: the normalization of heterosexual *institutions* that organize sexuality and reproduction, of heterosexual *identities* as discourses and practices that take heterosexuality for granted and mark LGBTQ identities as "other," and of phallocentric, goal-oriented, penetrative sexual practices. As Elia (2003) summarizes, "a specific brand of heterosexual relationship … has been promoted as the ultimate relational form at the expense of others who neither believe in nor practice such idealized relationships" (p. 61). Burgess (2005) notes that it is "on display every day in public spaces" (p. 27).

   In addition to law, custom, religion, and popular culture, sexology – and now sexual medicine – bolsters these norms through the construction and validation of what Nicolson (1993) has termed the *biological, coital*, and *orgasmic imperatives*, which normalize and essentialize reproductive, genital heterosex. These understandings of sexuality are also gendered through what Hollway (1984) termed the "male sex drive," "have/hold," and "permissive" discourses that permeate sexology and popular thought.[2]

A central theme of this book is that the achievement of "normal" heterosexuality is often hard work. Duncombe and Marsden (1996) have labelled this interpersonal labour a form of "sex work," while Harvey and Gill (2011) more lightly term emotional and sexual labour within a personal relationship as "intimate entrepreneurship" (p. 3).[3] Interpersonal sex work is ultimately connected to what Giddens (1991) refers to as 'the reflexive project of the self,' once imagined through self-help, but now, I would argue, through the pharmaceutical maximization of one's human potential. Increasingly, successful heterosexuality depends on pharmaceutical agents, from oral contraceptive pills, to the HPV vaccine, to hormone replacement therapy (see Polzer & Knabe, 2012). While trans* identities are often singled out for being technologically mediated, the gender identity of the middle-class, gender-conforming subject also might be achieved through technological interventions such as drugs (including hormones), chemical products, and surgeries. I make this point not in the spirit of condemning technological mediation or the work associated with identity formation, but rather to note its role in the most hegemonic of identities.

It is important to keep in mind that heteronormativity has been and continues to be consciously challenged and resisted through means other than embracing or rejecting technologies. Social movements in the 1970s that culminated in what is known as the "sexual revolution" were key in deconstructing and challenging heteronormative sex, advocating coming out as gay, lesbian, or bisexual, embracing political lesbianism, or resisting within heterosexual relationships. Anne Koedt's "The Myth of the Vaginal Orgasm" (1973) and Shere Hite's report on female sexuality (1976) exposed misunderstandings about female sexual pleasure and questioned the relegation of clitoral stimulation as "foreplay." Radical feminists named penetration as an act of patriarchal violence (see, for example, Dworkin, 1987), whereas others chose to reconceptualize and rename penetration in ways that did not position men as active doers of the act and women as passive recipients (for example, as "enclosure"; see Hite, 1976, p. 12).

In the second wave of feminism, there was a tendency, with examples such as Adrienne Rich's attack on "compulsory heterosexuality" (1980), to identify heterosexual practices with the oppressiveness of heterosexuality as an institution. In the 1990s, however, this conflation was challenged by feminists who attempted to disentangle heterosexual practices from the wider institution of heterosexuality (see, for example, (Jackson, 1999; Richardson, 1996; Smart, 1996). The feminist "sex wars" of this time stemmed from the polemic in feminist scholarship, activism, and praxis about how best to interpret and approach power and pleasure in the heterosexual context. Debates centred on whether sexualities both inside and outside the "charmed circle" (Rubin, 1984) of matrimonially based heterosexual reproduction should be conceived of as "primarily dangerous or should be embraced as pleasurable" (Vance, 1984, p. 7).

Increasingly, scholarship attempts to emphasize that heterosexuality (like any sexual identity) is "not a monolithic entity" (Jackson, 1999, p. 129); rather, "self formation is a variable process" (Jackson, 2006, p. 116). To capture such nuances, Rubin (1984, p. 280) discusses "hierarchies of sexual value" within heterosexuality where, for example, kink sex or sex in public is still heavily stigmatized. Heterosex might be transgressed non-deliberately or subverted, meaning a "reflexive undermining of heteronormativity that can produce challenges to or shifts in the norm, even if these do not appear to be radical" (Beasley, Brook, & Holmes, 2012, p. 5). Gender variation and fluidity also disrupt the strict correlation between heterosexuality and normativity. As queer theorists destabilize binaries of sex, gender, and sexuality, they argue that heterosexuality must be assessed in a more "context specific" light (p. 91). And yet, others still remind us that, despite more fluid sexual practices and theorizations, we must not lose sight of the "mundane" aspects of sex (Plummer, 2007) and the influence of material factors shaping and limiting sexual options and choices (Jackson, 1999).

Also relevant to this book, heteronormativity might not have "relinquished its hegemonic hold" on same-sex sexuality (Richardson, 1996, p. 3), as some argue that "there is no total escape from framing of the heterosexual desire within a social order where heterosexuality is so privileged" (Jackson, 1999, pp. 177–8). In other words, same-sex sexuality might not lie completely outside heterosexual hegemony. Moreover, we might need to move beyond the concept of "compulsory heterosexuality" (Rich, 1980, p. 632) to think about what Potts (2002) has termed "compulsory sex[uality]" (p. 56) or what Przybylo (2011) calls "sexuosociety" (p. 446). Although same-sex and queer sexualities increasingly are embraced in the mainstream, there is an assumption, also evident in feminist literature, that all people have the desire to be sexual, and that realizing sexual desire through orgasm completes straight *or* LGBTQ subjects in some ontological sense. The "over-investment" in sexuality "burdens sexuality with new expectations" (Foucault, 1979, quoted in Tyler, 2004, p. 99). Indeed, the rising asexuality movement, a grass-roots movement of young people in the West, challenges the notion that romantic or sexual relationships and interactions are important to everyone (Fahs, 2010).

When theorizing about heterosexuality from a feminist perspective, some authors draw on post-structuralist notions of power, validating women's ability to reshape or reinscribe heterosexual activities with new meanings and agency, especially at the micro level (Hollway, 1984; Smart, 1996). Others warn that we should be wary of grasping too readily this optimistic possibility of heterosexual empowerment, as the micro-politics of sexual relationships are deeply entwined with the "institutionalized gender inequalities of power" (Duncombe & Marsden, 1996, p. 221). As Jackson (1999) bluntly states, "our capacity to undo gender and heterosexuality is constrained by the structural inequalities which sustain them" (p. 181). I first and foremost set out to explore the nuances of the polemic that had formed regarding the medicalization and treatment of women's sexual problems. As one who finds value in both of the above theorizations of sexuality and power, however, and does not view them as entirely at odds, I was also curious to see what light these case studies of (mainly heterosexual) women who do not, cannot, or will not meet (mainly hetero) sexual norms for a variety of reasons, might shed on this theoretical polemic.

## The Structure of the Book

In this book I investigate this dynamic sexual pharmaceutical era in relation to original empirical data, and develop distinctive arguments that contribute to feminist, sociological scholarship on sex and medicine in the following ways. First, my research reminds us of the pervasiveness of the medicalization of heterosex and that working to achieve heterosexual norms without a drug is an established pattern for women that predates recent developments in sexual medicine and the sexual pharmaceutical industry. Second, it adds to the very small body of existing literature that argues that "sex work" occurs in personal, supposedly unpaid, non-commercial sexual relationships, with women's work outweighing men's in heterosexual relationships (Duncombe & Marsden, 1996). Third, I examine the literature on whether challenging or "queering" sexual norms in the context of heterosex, or refuting sexual relationships all together, transgresses or subverts hegemonic power relations.

In Chapter 1, "The Rise and Decline of Big Pharma's 'Sexual Revolu-tion,'" I outline the search for a sexual enhancement drug for women following the commercial success of Viagra. Despite their clear goals of profit and career expansion, drug companies (and the researchers and clinicians they sponsor) clothe this search in the rhetoric of female sex-ual empowerment. But so far every attempt to find a safe and effective magic-bullet cure for women's sexual problems has failed. In part this failure stems from the flaws inherent in the frameworks of sexuality on which these drugs are based. It is also due to the ways medicalized frameworks have been challenged by doctors within sexual medicine, as well as by health practitioners, scholars, and activists outside sexual medicine.

Chapter 2, "Treating Women's Sexual Pain: Biomedicalized, Demedi-calized, and Do-It-Yourself Approaches," critically examines treatments for sexual pain, including sexual pharmaceuticals, desensitization tech-niques, and do-it-yourself, inexpensive, approaches that have been adopted at the grassroots level. Since no magic-bullet cure for wom-en's lack of sexual desire, arousal, and orgasm has been found, drug companies and those they fund have turned their attention to treating women's sexual pain with more sophisticated biomedical technolo-gies. At the same time, as described by the lay and professional women I interviewed and observed, health professionals have adopted inno-vative, patient-led desensitization strategies. I argue that (bio)medi-calization, demedicalization, and grassroots strategies share more in common than is often assumed. Among other aspects, all are oriented towards the endpoint of restoring penetrative sex. In addition, self-help literature and groups are often dedicated to sharing biomedical information, and biomedical treatments are often remarkably low-tech, sharing some similarities (as well as differences) with grassroots femi-nist consciousness-raising techniques.

In Chapter 3, "The Limits of Normative Heterosex," I argue that the psycho-social and interpersonal context of sexual activity is central to women's experiences and judgment of sexual problems. When hetero-sexual women do not or cannot conform to one or more of the expecta-tions of normative heterosexuality, they have a particularly intense and conscious awareness of heterosexual standards, of the value afforded them, and, in many cases, of their coercive power. When reflecting on early and/or adult heterosex, participants in this study detailed gender-based relationship inequalities, violence, and coercion matter-of-factly, often expressing disappointment with the limited repertoire that normative heterosex demands. Their awareness of these limits, and their resignation to them, might indicate some of the paradoxes of this so-called post-feminist age.

Chapter 4, "Sex Work: A Labour of Love," considers the sexual division of relationship-based "sex work," which has been particularly onerous for women following the liberalization, commodification, and (re)medicalization of sex in the mid- to late twentieth century. The majority of women in this study were not diagnosed with FSD. However, most of this predominantly urban, middle-class sample spent time and energy on improving their perceived sexual difficulties as advised by a range of medical and non-medical sex experts. As varied as were the approaches taken by these women, the overall goal of most therapies was to hone skills such as discipline, concentration, and focus in order to alter their response to heteronormative sex. In many cases, practitioners and their clients had to negotiate the paradox of working towards sexual pleasure in cases where sex work was painful, uncomfortable, and distinctly non-pleasurable.

In Chapter 5, "Refusing Heteronormative Sex Work," I argue that not every woman works to achieve sexual desire, arousal, orgasm, and/or penetration. I discuss possible strategies for refusing the labour of love, including the option of changing one's sex life, rather than working on sex – for example, "queering" the normative sexual script or deprioritizing sex altogether and celebrating the non-sexual aspects of life. Highlighting the influence of material pressures on shaping women's sexual choices, for the most part, is that women who depended on their partners financially and/or had children were more hesitant about opting out of sex work.

In Chapter 6, "A Woman's Work Is Never Done," I summarize my empirical findings and connect the findings on (bio)medicalization, heteronormativity, and the reciprocal relationship between these two social processes. Big Pharma's "second sexual revolution" for women has not taken off the way industry hopefuls had intended, in part because sexual problems are shaped by a wealth of socio-political and interpersonal determinants that cannot be addressed by swallowing a pill. Even so, heterosexual women are encouraged and impelled to judge their sexuality in relation to the heterosexual gold standard of frequent intercourse ending in orgasm, and to analyse, monitor, and manage their and their partner's sexual experiences accordingly. Although some aspects of sex work are experienced as enjoyable and empowering, others are perceived of as uncomfortable, non-pleasurable, and expensive. These findings highlight existing inequalities and norms in heterosexual relationships that continue to shape many women's sexual experiences. Although an increasing number of sexual identities and practices have been depathologized, and positive portrayals of active sexuality are more abundant, these trends have been paralleled by new standards, anxieties, and forms of scrutiny. Despite social, commercial, and medical pressures, however, some women refuse to work towards heterosexual standards, opting instead to write their own rules. Since many have faced material consequences as a result (and others have conformed to sex work for fear of material outcomes), the institution of heterosexuality seems to be destabilized, only to be reinforced, when women refuse the "labour of love."

Finally, in the Epilogue, "The Sexual Pharmaceutical Industry and Its Discontents," I consider how the sexual pharmaceutical industry is both growing and showing signs of fatigue. As the medicalization of sex faces a broad, interdisciplinary critique, the industry and the doctors it funds are developing new ways to defend their efforts. I also set out emerging questions for feminist academic inquiry.

# 1 The Rise and Decline of Big Pharma's "Sexual Revolution"

When Pfizer Inc. launched Viagra as a "miracle drug" for the treatment of erectile dysfunction (ED) in 1998, speculation about a "second sexual revolution," as the *New York Times* dubbed this development, was almost immediate (Hitt, 2000). By Viagra's tenth anniversary, its revolutionary status was apparently confirmed, with major newspapers around the world celebrating "the little blue pill" that launched the "second sexual revolution."

It was not long before drug companies and the scientists and doctors they sponsor turned their attention to developing a sexual pharmaceutical for women. Since the launch of Viagra, the media has been rife with speculation that, as supposedly was the case with the oral contraceptive pill in the late 1960s, a pill could be pivotal in revolutionizing sex for women. As a journalist for *Vogue* magazine boldly stated, "In the first [sexual revolution], women asserted their rights to a fulfilling sex life ..., in the second, enterprising medics and entrepreneurs are working hard to deliver it" (Hutton, 2003, p. 1).

From the vantage point of a decade and a half after the approval of Viagra, in this chapter I sketch the male sexual pharmaceutical market and Viagra's fragile position as the top-grossing and most popular sexual pharmaceutical for men. I then shift the focus to drug industry attempts to develop a pharmaceutical sexual revolution for women, introducing the cast of characters who have touted sexual pharmaceuticals as solving women's sexual problems, while so clearly motivated by career success, profit, and fame. I explain why sexual pharmaceuticals for women thus far have failed, and the role dissidents in the medical profession and various scholars and activists have played in challenging these developments. While this chapter sets the stage for

understanding a polemic that has informed the critique of the medicalization of sexual "function" and "dysfunction," the rest of the book
deals with the much more ordinary and less often discussed topics of
how heterosexual women in North America view the origins of their
perceived sexual problems, what they do to solve, deal with, move
past, transgress, or subvert them in everyday life, and how intersecting aspects of identity such as race, class, and sexuality influence their
perceptions and experiences.

## The Sexual Pharmaceutical "Revolution" for Men

As Meika Loe (2004a) documents in *The Rise of Viagra: How A Little
Blue Pill Changed Sex in America,* the Viagra "revolution" was sparked,
according to public relations mythology, by an accidental discovery.
When Pfizer Inc. tested sildenafil citrate in clinical trials as a treatment
for angina, its erection-enhancing properties were an unexpected side
effect. Pfizer seized on this accidental opportunity, branding the drug
Viagra – the name a mix of vigour and Niagara – and the "disorder"
of "erectile dysfunction" that Viagra would treat. By 2003 Viagra had
reached the blockbuster success of Prozac, spawning copycat drugs
such as Cialis, Levitra, Staxyn, and Stendra.[1] In the process, Pfizer spent
more money than ever before on drug advertising to reach a wider,
albeit mainly white, heterosexual, gender-normative audience. Most
surprising was the appearance of former US presidential candidate Bob
Dole as a spokesperson for Viagra.

  Yet it is now clear that Viagra is in no way a panacea for men's sexual
problems. Conservative estimates are that more than one-third of Viagra
prescriptions are not refilled (Hwancheol, Kwanjin, Soo-Woong, &
Jae-Seung, 2004; Klotz, Mathers, Klotz, & Sommer, 2005). As noted in
an article in the *Journal of the American Medical Association* titled "Some
Men Who Take Viagra Die: Why?" (Mitka, 2000), in the first year of its
release, there were 49 deaths from heart failure per one million Viagra
users (for a total of 564 deaths). The manufacturer thus had to add a
mandatory warning label about the contraindications of heart conditions and Viagra. From its early days, there were also concerns that
Viagra might cause vision loss. A 2010 US Food and Drug Administration (FDA) audit of Viagra's side effects found that Pfizer had "failed
to submit reports of vision loss associated with Viagra in a timely fashion or downgraded the seriousness of those reports even though they
involved 'blindness' and 'visual acuity loss/reduction" (Edwards,

2010, para. 1). As well, although many partners of Viagra users might be thrilled with the sexual opportunities the drug affords, many others are not (Loe, 2004b; Potts, Gavey, Grace, & Vares, 2003). Complaints include pressure to be sexually "on" once a partner pops this expensive pill, an increased incidence of coerced sex, and the reinstatement of penetrative sex as the only option on the sexual menu, particularly later in life. Finally, although Viagra offers a short-term quick fix for erectile problems, it does not address premature ejaculation or low desire (Loe, 2004a).

Not surprisingly, movements are afoot to capitalize on the potential market for treating men's low sexual desire. Men's sexual problems are now being reframed as testosterone deficiency treatable by a testosterone gel. In 2011 Abbott Laboratories, the maker of AndroGel, a testosterone drug, launched a Canadian website and sponsored a week-long advertisement (which did not mention the drug) in the *Globe and Mail* newspaper for a "disease awareness" campaign highlighting "low T," or low testosterone. The sexy ad emphasized the use of testosterone as a therapy for low sexual desire in men with captions such as "Has He Lost That Loving Feeling?" A slick ninety-second ad for AndroGel also aired on television during the 2012 Summer Olympic Games depicting fit, muscular bodies, using imagery of "many things rising," and repeating words such as "big" and "raises" (Dubowitz, Puretz, and Fugh-Berman, 2012, para. 3).

By 2013 sales of AndroGel, at US$874 million, had almost surpassed those of Viagra. Since generic versions will be allowed as of 2015, Abbott Laboratories has attempted to boost its brand loyalty with a "Got Low T?" campaign published in newspapers across North America, Europe, and Australia. The ads direct readers to a website that lists the supposed symptoms of "Low T": "unwanted body changes," "reduced sex drive," "difficulty maintaining an erection" and "decreased energy."[2] There, visitors can take a short quiz assessing whether they have "Low T." If they answer "yes" to either of the questions, "do you have a decrease in libido (sex drive)?" and "are your erections less strong?" they are encouraged to "talk to your doctor." The site even offers to email the results to visitors, who then can print them and bring them to their next doctor's appointment. Significantly, the "Got Low T?" site also speaks directly to assumed heterosexual female partners, even including a page titled "tips for talking to him," calling on women to "offer to accompany him to the doctor's office" and to "help him recognize his symptoms may be caused by a medical condition."

Meanwhile, despite such competition, Pfizer's Viagra remains the top-grossing and best-known sexual pharmaceutical on the market. Eventually, however, the expiration of Pfizer's patent will leave the company vulnerable to competition from generic manufacturers that could offer the same substance at a lower price. Indeed, Teva Pharmaceuticals managed some years ago to gain tentative approval from the FDA to market a generic version of Viagra, but in March 2010 Pfizer sued Teva for patent infringement. Using its recent research into the effects of sildenafil citrate on children with pulmonary hypertension as the reason for the importance of its original patent, Pfizer has ensured that no generic sildenafil citrate can be produced in the United States until 2020 (Viagra Patent Expiration Extended to 2020, 2013, para. 3). It has also been successful in securing a second patent, referred to in the industry as a "method-of-treatment" patent, until 2019, that ensures that Pfizer will be the only company that is able to market its drug as a treatment for ED. Nevertheless, in Canada, the Supreme Court of Canada ruled in favour of Teva's claim to the rights to produce a generic version ("Viagra patent tossed out by the Supreme Court," 2012), and Pfizer's patent expired in the European Union on 21 June 21 2013 (Palmer, 2013).

### Creating the Market for Sexual Pharmaceuticals for Women

It was not long after the "happy accident" of Viagra's discovery that scientists, doctors, and the drug companies that fund them began a tireless search for a "pink" Viagra for women that would expand the market for sexual pharmaceuticals by an estimated US$1.7 billion (Hartley, 2006). Indeed, the search for a sexual enhancement drug for women was not born out of revolutionary ideas about women and sexuality, but rather of a commercial partnership between physicians and drug companies. In one of the most heavily critiqued instances of what drug industry insiders term "condition branding" (Angelmar, Angelmar, & Kane, 2007) and critics refer to as "disease mongering" (Moynihan, 2003; Tiefer, 2006b), pharmaceutical companies and the medics they fund have busied themselves creating a market of women labelled as having "female sexual dysfunction" (FSD). In the process, they ignored social factors shaping women's experience, and portrayed FSD as a physiological disorder – the complex female counterpart to ED, although the definition included not only dysfunctional arousal, but also desire, orgasm, and pain (Basson, Berman, Burnett, Derogatis, Ferguson, et al., 2001).

The statistic that 43 per cent of women suffer from FSD has been cited more than a thousand times (Moynihan, 2003; Moynihan & Mintzes, 2010). Yet this figure is based on a gross misinterpretation of the results of a national survey of over 3,000 Americans, intended as an update to Kinsey's work, on the post-HIV sexual climate of the United States and published in the early 1990s (Laumann, Gagnon, Michael, & Michaels, 1994). Among other things, the survey asked a series of questions about whether women had experienced any sexual difficulties in the past year – for example, if they lacked interest in sex, felt anxious about their sexual performance, had trouble with lubrication, failed to orgasm, came to orgasm too quickly, or experienced pain with intercourse. The 43 per cent statistic came from assuming that an answer of "yes" to any one of these questions was grounds for categorizing the respondent as having FSD. When Viagra was introduced, this particular part of the survey was published in the *Journal of the American Medical Association* with a recommendation that therapies be developed for women with sexual dysfunction (Laumann, Paik, & Rosen, 1999). Later it was revealed that two of the authors, Edward Laumann and Ray Rosen, had financial ties to Pfizer. Laumann has since denounced this interpretation of the survey results, claiming that the idea to ask questions on sexual difficulties and then to interpret "yes" answers as evidence of dysfunction, came from co-author Rosen, a psychologist who has collaborated with drug companies since the initial success of Viagra.

Although a vast network of Pharma-funded physicians from around the world has contributed to positioning FSD as a serious medical condition and branding medical attention to this diagnosis as a step towards women's sexual equality and empowerment, among the best known are Dr Irwin Goldstein and Dr Jennifer Berman (along with her sister, Laura Berman). The careers of these particular doctors might represent an extreme, but they are nonetheless symbolic of emerging trends in the increasingly biomedicalized and commercialized world of health care.

Before the FDA even approved Viagra, Goldstein, a urologist and director of Boston University's Institute for Sexual Medicine, began efforts to "pre-organize" the FSD market (Fishman, 2004) with the publication of an article in the *Urology Times* titled "New Field Could Open for Urologists: Female Sexual Dysfunction" (Goldstein, 1997). He had already established himself as an expert in male sexual dysfunction in the 1980s (Krane, Siroky, and Goldstein, 1983). As Tiefer (2001) relates, in the early days of Viagra, Goldstein organized, chaired, and attended a number of key meetings on FSD funded by the drug industry. In 1997 he planned The Cape Cod Meeting, the first of many meetings dedicated solely to FSD. Only drug companies and sex researchers connected to the drug industry were invited. In 1998 nineteen international sexual health specialists – all but one with professional links to pharmaceutical companies, including Pfizer – were included in Goldstein's International Consensus Development Conference, whose purpose was to create a consensus document on the FSD diagnosis. In 1999, as another way of institutionalizing FSD, Goldstein began to host annual conferences on continuing medical education (CME) ( Fishman, 2004; Hartley & Tiefer, 2003). Billed as educational, in 2001 these conferences spawned the professional organization later named the International Society for the Study of Women's Sexual Health. Since 2005, Goldstein has been editor in chief of the *Journal of Sexual Medicine*, now seen as the most influential publication in sexual medicine. In 2006 he co-edited the definitive textbook on FSD (Goldstein, Meston, Davis, & Traish, 2006), according him a unique degree of influence on the direction of sexual dysfunction research and clinical practice.

The year before the release of Viagra, Jennifer Berman became the first doctor to publish a pilot study on the drug's effects on women with arousal and orgasm difficulties. Pfizer took note of this young doctor and awarded her its Scholar of Urology Award in 1998. That same year she was offered the position of co-directing the Boston University Women's Sexual Health Clinic with Goldstein. She brought her sex therapist sister Laura on board, and since then the two have been an unstoppable team. In 2000 the two Bermans left Boston to operate the female sexual medicine centre at the University of California, Los Angeles (UCLA), then, in 2005, they parted ways professionally. In the meantime, they co-chaired several annual Women's Sexual Health State of the Art CME conferences at UCLA and Northwestern University, where Laura Berman holds an academic appointment. These CME conferences were funded by unrestricted educational grants from pharmaceutical companies and focused mainly on information about the physiological causes and medical treatment of FSD (Fishman, 2004).

The Bermans are best known, however, for using the media, rather than traditional academic channels, to build the FSD brand. The attractive, blond, blue-eyed sister team has appeared on television talk shows such as *Good Morning America, Larry King Live, 48 Hours,* and *The Oprah Winfrey Show.* They have been interviewed in every major women's magazine, including *Vogue, Elle,* and *Glamour.* Widely recognized as "celebrity doctors," for three years they hosted an FSD-related television talk show titled *Berman and Berman* for the Discovery Health Channel. Laura Berman went on to host a radio talk show on Oprah Radio titled *Better in Bed With Dr. Berman,* which then became a Harpo Productions television talk show featured on Oprah's OWN network. To date, the sisters have co-authored two best-selling books on FSD: *For Women Only: A Revolutionary Guide to Overcoming Sexual Dysfunction and Reclaiming Your Sex Life* (with Elizabeth Bulmiller, 2001) and *Secrets of the Sexually Satisfied Woman: Ten Keys to Unlocking Ultimate Sexual Pleasure* (with Alice Schweiger, 2006). Laura Berman has also published several solo-authored books (Berman 2006; 2008; 2009; 2010b; 2010c; 2011).

In 2005 the Bermans closed down the UCLA centre, crossing the increasingly thin line from academic sexual medicine to the private, commercial sector. Laura left first to open a treatment clinic in Chicago. Jennifer left the next year to open a private "boutique practice, outside of academia" (O'Connor, 2005, para. 52) in Beverly Hills. These clinics were meant to be prototypes of a future chain of sexual medicine clinics that would offer medical, psychological, urogynecologic, and hormonal evaluations and treatments, in addition to nutrition, fitness, and "successful aging" programs.

Jennifer Berman's clinic blends sex therapy with highly medicalized forms of assessment and treatment, including the use of equipment designed to assess "vagina elasticity," "vaginal pH," "clitoral and labial sensation," and "pelvic blood flow." Her website (www.bermansexual health.com) does not advertise a pricelist, but suggests an in-person or over-the-telephone consultation to discuss pricing. As seen in the documentary *Orgasm Inc: The Strange Science of Female Pleasure* (Canner, 2011), when filmmaker Liz Canner was given the full in-house assessment, her bill totalled US$1,500, which did not include treatment. In the film, the camera pans to a sign on the clinic entry door that reads "Please be aware the Berman Center does not accept insurance." Below, it states "Insurance typically does not cover the services we provide."

And yet the vanguards of this sexual pharmaceutical industry position their efforts explicitly in feminist and revolutionary terms. Goldstein has been quoted as saying, "Our knowledge of sexual health is in revolutionary mode" (in Hitt, 2000, para. 6). Both Bermans are vocal in their view that medical attention to treating FSD is analogous to promoting women's rights to sexual pleasure. Laura Berman refers to their work as promoting a "grassroots movement" in sexual health (O'Connor, 2005, para. 39). The stated goal of one of Berman and Berman's best-selling books summarizes this approach. Mirroring the language of feminist health collectives, they write:

> Our goal in this books is to arm women with the information they need about their bodies ... Our hope is that women will take this book to their doctors, give it to their partners, or share it with other women. It is written without jargon, for women, by women. Clearly the options will continue to grow as more research is done in the field, and it is also our plan to update women with the latest information. We are in a era of women's sexual health – perhaps feminism's next frontier ... It is time for women to receive the same attention as men, and to demand treatment, not only for pain, but to increase their sexual pleasure. (Berman et al. 2001, p. xv1)

Elsewhere, Jennifer Berman refers to herself as a "pioneer," stating, "I was probably the first doctor to give [Viagra] to women" (O'Connor, 2005, para. 22). Media reports also bolster this view of the sister team as leaders of a sexual revolution, with titles such as "Sisters are doing it for themselves" (Berens, 2001) and "Our bodies, ourselves" (O'Connor, 2005, para. 20). Unlike feminist understandings of sexuality, however, the Bermans fear that recognizing social factors as potentially inhibiting sexual pleasure might delegitimize the field of sexual medicine. They write: "It is still shocking for us to hear how many doctors, female as well as male, tell their female patients that their problems are emotional, relational, due to fatigue from child rearing or their busy jobs, and that they should take care of their problems on their own" (Berman et al., 2001, p. xiii).

Doctors connected to the medicalization of women's sexual problems have been loathe to admit how much they have earned as a result of related pharmaceutical funding. In 2005 a journalist for the *Los Angeles Times* asked Jennifer Berman how much she earned as a consultant for Pfizer, Vivus, Cellegy, Bayer, Eli Lilly, and Proctor & Gamble. She avoided the question, but stated that, like other urologists, she is frequently offered ski trips, first-class plane tickets, and other forms of "wining and dining." She adamantly denied having taken any vacation offers, but conceded, "[e]very night you're out – one night with Bayer, the next night with Pfizer." She also revealed that she is paid between US$10,000 and $75,000 for media endorsements of products such as

Viagra, explaining that, "[o]nce you deal with the marketing side …, there's usually more resources" (quoted in O'Connor, 2005, para. 27). This same article revealed that the sisters earned more than US$1 million for the TV show *Berman and Berman*.

Cracks have formed, however, in the original team of sexual medicine specialists who were once united in their search for the perfect sex drug for women. In an interview, Jennifer Berman said she left the UCLA clinic because her colleagues were "jealous" and "mean" about her success (O'Connor, 2005, para. 4). Even long-time mentor Irwin Goldstein has stated publicly that the Bermans have gone too far in their commercialized approach. Of Jennifer Berman, his former colleague, he commented to a reporter, "Jennifer didn't want to be in our world. I presume her world may be more lucrative" (quoted in O'Connor, 2005, para. 19). Yet Goldstein, too, left Boston University's Institute for Sexual Medicine in 2005 in search of a more supportive academic environment in which to practise sexual medicine. After a year and a half, he ended up at Alvarado Hospital in San Diego, California. The hospital was forced into sale after several years of legal and financial problems, but was eventually purchased by a former colleague of Goldstein's. He has now established a sexual medicine program that he hopes will be a destination for people seeking treatment or doing research in sexual medicine (Darcé, 2007). In any event, new thought leaders, such as Michael Krychman and Sheryl A. Kingsberg (2013), have emerged in the race to find a sexual pharmaceutical drug for women.

**The Anticlimax**

Fifteen years after the approval of Viagra and the attending cries of revolution, it seems that the pharmaceutical sexual revolution for women has yet to take off in the way the drug industry and its connected physicians had hoped. Despite major efforts, drug companies and the researchers they fund have failed to find a one-size-fits-all drug with any meaningful benefit to solving women's sexual problems beyond a placebo in clinical trials. Several drugs aimed at women are still in the pipeline. In the meantime, thought leaders associated with Big Pharma can only prescribe drugs "off-label," endorse nutriceuticals, or, as I examine in Chapter 2, treat sexual pain issues.

As Loe (2004a) documents, following the perceived success of Viagra as a treatment for men's ED, researchers advocated a vascular or blood-flow approach to managing FSD. This understanding was inspired by a hydraulic model of sexual functioning, the same kind of framework researchers used in studying men's erectile difficulties. When touting a vascular approach, their focus was on female sexual arousal disorder (FSAD), a subset of FSD, which could most logically be treated by a vascular drug. For instance, in their presentations at the Boston conference in 1999, members of the original Boston group made frequent reference to terms such as "vaginal compliance" and "genital response" and used labels such as "vaginal engorgement insufficiency" and "clitoral erectile insufficiency" (Loe, 2004a, p. 66). In 2000 Goldstein espoused the logic of the vascular model in a *New York Times* article, stating, "I am an engineer ... I can apply the principles of hydraulics to these problems. I can utilize medical strategies to assess, diagnose, and manipulate things that are not so straightforward in psychiatry" (quoted in Hitt, 2000, para. 10). In fact, Goldstein collaborated with Boston University's department of aerospace engineering in formulating his theories on the vascular elements of women's sexual arousal problems.[3] Viagra itself was the most obvious choice as a vascular drug for women, but even Pfizer-funded studies could not prove any meaningful benefit from the drug for women's sexual arousal (Basson, McInnes, Smith, Hodgson, & Koppiker, 2002).

The vascular approach did not lead to the approval of a drug for the treatment for FSD, but it did inspire the FDA-approved Eros clitoral therapy *device* (CTD), which is thought to enhance blood flow to the clitoris (see Fishman and Mamo, 2001).[4] Manufacturers of the Eros CTD describe it as "designed to treat forms of FSD caused by inadequate blood flow to the genitalia providing suction directly to the clitoris, causing engorgement." Although "the device seems to resemble an over-the-counter sex toy in shape and function, it is carefully constructed as a device for 'treatment' rather than for 'pleasure'" (Fishman and Mamo, 2001, p. 188). It also costs US$359. Instructions for the device tell users that it is not meant to replace intercourse as the main event during sex, but is recommended for use "alone" or as "part of foreplay." Although sexual medicine specialists frequently prescribe the device, a medicalized sex toy is hardly the cure-all that the drug industry and industry-funded physicians had hoped for.

Not satisfied with the limited success of the vascular model in leading to a blockbuster drug, in 2000 the Boston group began to consider the possibility that women's sexual difficulties should be treated as hormonal problems. At a conference session on "Desire, Arousal, and Testosterone," Goldstein told the audience that he regularly prescribes dehydroepiandrosterone (DHEA), an over-the-counter supplement linked to testosterone production. He reported, "[a]ll I can tell you is what I tell my patients – it's like gas in a car. You can't drive unless you have gas. Testosterone is the gas" (quoted in Loe, 2004a, p. 150). Goldstein's wife Sue also gave a talk on the benefits of using DHEA based on her own experiences with the supplement.

It was no accident that 2000 was the year of "desire" and "hormones" in the world of sexual medicine. The same year, publicity began to emerge about Intrinsa, a testosterone patch developed by Procter & Gamble for the treatment of hypoactive sexual desire disorder (HSDD). Soon after the announcement of phase-two clinical trials of Intrinsa, a conference titled "Androgen Deficiency in Women: Definition, Diagnosis, and Classification" was announced. The conference was sponsored by "unrestricted educational grants" from a number of pharmaceutical companies, all with testosterone products in the pipeline. Just months before the FDA hearing on the drug, Laura Berman wrote an op-ed for the *Chicago Sun-Times* titled "Not in the mood? Now there's a patch" (Berman, 2004).

Intrinsa was denied FDA approval in 2004, with the FDA noting a high placebo effect in clinical trial participants. Aside from the fact that "sexually satisfying events," a subjective measurement, rose only from three to four per month, safety was the main concern. According to the FDA, Proctor & Gamble did not have an adequate post-approval surveillance plan; as well, although Intrinsa is a testosterone patch, Proctor & Gamble tested it only on women already taking estrogen. To date, combined estrogen and testosterone therapy remains medically controversial, as little research has been done to investigate its long-term effects on women, especially those in their twenties and thirties (Basson, 2008). Intrinsa was approved in the European Union for pre-menopausal women who had undergone a hysterectomy, but its maker has withdrawn it from the market, suggesting either a lack of popularity or a high rate of adverse events. LibiGel, a testosterone gel for women to be applied to the arm daily and currently under phase-three clinical trials, is being marketed as a "revolutionary step forward in improving women's female sexual health."[5]

In 2010 the media buzzed with hype that the "pink" Viagra had been discovered at last in the form of a brain drug, Flibanserin, made by German company Boehringer Ingelheim (BI). The drug was heralded as a Viagra equivalent for women even though it was designed to target the brain, not blood flow, and desire, not arousal.[6] It also would have to be taken daily. As one of its main consultants, BI hired Irwin Goldstein, the same doctor who espoused the view that testosterone therapy was *the* answer for women's sexual woes. He then framed Flibanserin as *the* key to women's sexual enjoyment; as he told a reporter for *San Diego Magazine,* Flibanserin "has enormous potential to be a life-changing sort of product" (Perkins, 2011, para. 8).

The story of Flibanserin is remarkably similar to Pfizer's story about the "accidental" discovery of Viagra (Loe, 2004a). Flibanserin was a failed anti-depressant that, according to its maker, unexpectedly improved sexual desire in clinical trials testing. As in the case of Viagra, there was nothing accidental about what happened next. In the same way that Pfizer carefully marketed Viagra as a medical cure for a "serious" (that is, physiological) disorder, BI organized medical conferences, press releases, and phone and webcasts about HSDD. Using the resources of a public relations firm skilled in condition branding, the "Sex, Brain, Body Campaign" was far slicker than the Intrinsa campaign, and came complete with a celebrity endorsement by former Playboy model and soap star Lisa Rhinna. The maker also funded a Discovery Health Channel documentary about HSDD.

As media hype leading up to Flibanserin's FDA trial mounted, public statements by spokespeople for Flibanserin suggested that nobody was sure exactly how or why this drug could possibly be effective. In an interview for *Vogue* magazine, Dr Anita Clayton, a psychiatrist at the University of Virginia who led the clinical trials, stated: "It presumably frees up the inhibitory effect of serotonin on desire" (quoted in Jetter, 2010, p. 209). Dr Michael Krychman, another of BI's paid researchers, was invited on to Laura Berman's radio talk show to speak about the drug, and gave a rather vague explanation of how it worked: "The main mechanism still remains to be elucidated, but the nature of the drug, what we know about it, is that it really acts centrally in the brain" (Berman, 2010a).

As I and other critics prepared to testify against Flibanserin at FDA approval hearings (see Cacchioni, 2010), it was clear to us that there was little evidence to support the notion that Flibanserin was indeed a life-changing product. Although the FDA denied approval of the drug on 18 June 2010, a 2013 article in *Formulary Journal,* a peer-reviewed "drug management journal for managed care and hospital decision makers," continued to discuss Flibanserin as an investigational treatment in phase three of research (Krychman & Kingsberg, 2013). The authors made no mention of the FDA's having denied approval of the drug or of the funding they had received from BI. In 2011 a company called Sprout purchased Flibanserin from BI. Claiming to have "new" trial data, Sprout then resubmitted Flibanserin to the FDA. In a press report, Sprout's chief operating officer claimed that, "with this study and other information included in our resubmission, Sprout believes that it has addressed the concerns raised by the FDA during its previous review (Grogan, 2013, para 7). Nevertheless the FDA once again denied approval.

In March 2013 Emotional Brain, a Dutch- and US-based company, applied to the FDA for approval of two drugs called Lybrido and Lybridos. The announcement sparked Irwin Goldstein to declare prematurely that "2013 is the year of the woman" (Landau, 2013, para 40). Emotional Brain claims that the drugs bridge the gap between mind and body that sexual medicine believes has complicated the search for a magic-bullet cure for women's sexual dysfunction. Each drug consists of a mint-flavoured outer coating of testosterone, which dissolves in the mouth. Then, in the case of Lybrido – said to be a cousin of Viagra – once the pill is swallowed, a secondary delayed substance is released, a molecule that Emotional Brain claims causes extra blood flow to the genitals, adding swelling and sensation and working with the testosterone to spark dopamine networks. Lybridos has the same outer coating of testosterone as Lybrido, but instead of an arousal agent, it releases buspirone, an anti-anxiety medication said to affect serotonin levels in the brain. The company testing these drugs says that women will need blood work to ascertain which drug is appropriate for their particular case of HSDD. Although it is still compiling the results of its initial clinical trials, the maker is confident the drugs eventually will receive FDA approval. In an interview with Dr Andrew Goldstein in the *New York Times*, the creators of Lybrido are concerned that, if anything, it might be too effective, potentially spurring bouts of "female excess" and "crazed binges of infidelity" – as Goldstein blatantly states, "[y]ou want the effects to be good but not too good" (Hodgekiss, 2013, para. 20).

Last but not least, in May 2012 Trimel Pharmaceuticals announced the enrolment of 240 patients in a phase-two study in the United States of Tefina, an intra-nasal gel formulation of testosterone, the first drug proposed to treat "anorgasmia" or "orgasmic dysfunction." Health Canada and Australian authorities have also approved clinical trials of the drug. The success of Tefina will be measured by "the increase in the occurrence of orgasm compared against baseline levels."[7] During a 21 November 2012 interview for the CBC Radio show *The Current*, when the Australian lead investigator, Dr Susan Davis, was asked about the safety of testosterone drugs as raised in the Intrinsa trial, she claimed there were "no androgen side effects" associated with Tefina, even though the clinical trials were hardly under way. Of critics and sceptics, she stated, "It is a sexist and inappropriate concept to say it's not an appropriate drug for women ... [M]aybe they [the critics] have a problem. Maybe they're frigid." Barbara Mintzes, an independent drug reviewer interviewed for the same show, pointed out that androgen drugs are always treated as category X drugs and, therefore, always contraindicated for pregnancy.

The search for a "pink" Viagra eventually might come full circle. In the lead-up to the Flibanserin FDA hearing, Pfizer announced that it had a sexuopharmaceutical for women in the pipeline, a drug it refers to in its pre-branded state as UK-414, 495. A British Pfizer scientist tested the drug on anesthetized rabbits that were dosed with ketamine, a veterinary aesthetic often used by humans as a recreational drug, and found that it might have blood-flow-enhancing properties. Nevertheless, Pfizer might simply be trying to keep its name in the race to find such a drug. And, not surprisingly, since the drug operates on a vascular model much like Viagra, Pfizer's public statements on its potential for women are accompanied by old quotes from Irwin Goldstein and the Bermans. There is a returned focus to FSAD, long forgotten amid the recent hype about drugs promising to treat HSDD. Despite media headlines, however, the drug has yet to be tested on women (Wayman, Baxter, Turner, Van Der Graaf, & Naylor, 2010).

In many countries, including Canada and the United States, restrictions on off-label prescribing were loosened in the 1990s (Conrad & Leiter, 2004). Thus, physicians in the field of sexual medicine now frequently prescribe Viagra, Levitra, Cialis, and testosterone replacements such as AndroGel and Testim for women with FSD, even though these drugs have not been approved for this diagnosis. A definitive medical textbook on FSD (Goldstein et al., 2006) recommends off-label drugs, prescribing testosterone for "low libido," estrogen for "diminished arousal," and "systemic agents that are dopamine agonists, such as bupropion," for "low libido, orgasmic function, and sexual function" (p. 746). Even though clinical research proving that Viagra is rarely an effective solution for most women's sexual problems (Basson et al., 2002), the Bermans have been known to boast that physicians can prescribe Viagra for women. In 2010, when one guest caller on their radio show commented, "I thought it was just for men," Jennifer Berman replied: "Well, you're gonna learn." The Bermans directly encourage women to take Viagra off-label in their best-selling books, stating in one book that "a vasodilator like Viagra or one of the other drugs like it (Cialis or Levitra) should be considered if you have low arousal, especially if your doctor thinks the problem may be caused by nerve damage, aging, lack of use, or hormonal deficiencies" (Berman et al., 2001, p. 110).[8]

Finally, although pharmaceutical companies cannot advertise the off-label use of drugs directly, Goldstein and the Bermans, like many doctors in the current medical climate, have found ways around this. The Bermans advertise Viagra and other sexual pharmaceuticals and their possible off-label uses on all their websites, including the seemingly non-commercially titled Network for Excellence in Women's Sexual Health,[9] which they use to publish the findings of clinical trials without peer review. They also endorse over-the-counter nutriceuticals that do not require FDA approval. Zestra, a mixture of "pure botanical oils," which the Bermans have endorsed on their websites and in television appearances on *The Dr. Oz Show*, is advertised as having been tested "in conformance with FDA standards" by "independent medical researchers" (Hartley, 2006). The original study was based on a sample of only twenty women, although clinical trials are now under way in several sites across the United States.

And yet it seems that the thorny issue of the effect continues to tarnish the findings of any randomized, controlled study of sexual enhancement agents for women. Bradford and Meston (2009) review 165 articles detailing clinical trials for FSD drugs of various kinds, and report that "our review of the available data from the literature indicates that statistically significant and often substantial placebo responses are not uncommon in the biomedical treatment of women's sexual dysfunction" (p. 175). "Not uncommon" is putting it lightly, given that the vast majority of research Bradford and Meston survey demonstrates this pattern. It seems likely that the very acts of enrolling in a study to improve sexual enjoyment, engaging in a protocol of regular sexual activity with a partner or masturbating, and taking the time to reflect on this experience might themselves be an aphrodisiac. In other words, prioritizing sexual activity (perhaps with expert licence to do so as a bonus), taking the time to think about how the activity makes one feel, and having the time, space, and forum for reflection on these feelings is likely a formula for improved sexual enjoyment.

## Challenging the Sexual Pharmaceutical Revolution

The sexual pharmaceutical "revolution" is not simply self-imploding; it has been weakened by sexual medicine specialists and other experts who question and complicate the strictly physiological approach advocated by physicians with strong links to industry funding. These professionals operate within a medicalized framework, albeit a far more cautious one. Even more challenging, as illustrated by the sources used in this chapter, the New View Campaign (most notably by Leonore Tiefer) in concert with some excellent journalists (Canner, 2011; Moynihan, 2003) have tracked the every move of drug companies, the physicians they hire, and the marketing techniques they deploy.

Rosemary Basson's work is exemplary of a certain degree of dissent that has taken place within sexual medicine. She was a general practitioner who noticed the frequency of her patients' complaints about sexual enjoyment and decided to specialize in sexual medicine before taking this career path was linked to lucrative industry funding. Basson pieced together her own fellowship without pay at the University of British Columbia, and was given a position in the sexual medicine unit of Vancouver General Hospital. This unit was still part of British Columbia's universal health care program, but was then poorly funded.

Along with Goldstein and the Bermans, Basson is a signatory to the consensus report on the FSD classification system (Basson et al., 2001), discussed below, and is an influential player in the field of sexual medicine's take on FSD. Pfizer paid Basson to determine the efficacy of Viagra for women, but her published conclusion was that the drug was not effective (Basson et al., 2002). She went on to publish numerous articles critiquing the Masters and Johnson sexual response model that forms the basis of much of sexual medicine's thinking about the mechanics of sexual response (Basson 2001a, 2001b, 2001c, 2002a, 2002b, 2002c, 2002d, 2005). Basson has proposed a different model of sexual response for women, arguing that women are more likely to experience desire or "excitement" *after* sexual stimulus, initiated upon a woman's urge for emotional intimacy or her partner's desire for sex. Her theory that women "very often, begin sexual experiences from a state of sexual neutrality" (Basson 2002d, p. 22), rather than pre-existing, independent sexual desire, was based initially solely on clinical observation, but was later tested through an informal questionnaire of forty-seven of her patients who complained of low sexual desire. Describing this cycle, she explains:

> When a woman senses a potential opportunity to be sexual with her part-ner, although she may not "need" to experience arousal and resolution for her own sexual well-being, she is nevertheless motivated to deliberately do whatever is necessary to facilitate a sexual interaction as she expects potential benefits that, though not strictly sexual, are very important. The increased emotional closeness, bonding, commitment, tolerance of each other's imperfections, and expectation of increased well-being of the partner all serve as highly valid motivational factors that activate the cycle. She moves from a state of sexual neutrality, to open mindedness or willingness to be receptive to stimuli, to a degree of sexual pleasure and arousal. A sense of sexual desire to continue the experience then follows. Subsequently she may experience higher arousal and possibly orgasmic release. If the emotional aspect of the interaction, as well as the physical aspect, is positive, intimacy is enhanced and the cycle strengthened. In contrast, the traditional "human sex response cycle" of Masters and John-son and Kaplan, depicts sexual desire as a spontaneous force that itself triggers sexual arousal. (Basson, 2001c, pp. 396–7)

Hayes (2011), in the first comprehensive review of scientific models of sexual response, endorses Basson's cycle. By contrast, the findings of a focus group study with eighty participants conducted by Graham, Sanders, Milhausen, & McBride (2004) suggest that, for some women, sexual interest sometimes precedes arousal and sometimes proceeds arousal. Reflective of the dialogue within sexual medicine, Basson has been critiqued by sexual medicine researchers, including Both and Everaerd (2002), also signatories to the FSD consensus report (Basson et al., 2001), who argue that Basson's cycle merely replaces one univer-salizing cycle with another.

On first glance this cycle can be interpreted as reinforcing biologi-cal essentialism, much like the "male sex drive" and "have/hold" dis-courses in sexology (Hollway, 1984). However, Basson's reference to "potential benefits, though not strictly sexual" is a testament to her consciousness of the wider context in which heterosex takes place. Her research and published work is evidence of her implicit awareness of "the social," but also the medical tendency to categorize social issues as individual, psychological, or interpersonal issues. For instance, her

female sexual response cycle describes a low incidence of "independent sexual desire" prior to stimulation as "normal" for women due
to a number of "stresses," which she interprets as "psychological factors." She states: "Many psychological factors negatively influence the
processing of sexual cues in the limbic centres. Included are non-sexual
distractions, feeling sexually substandard, past negative or painful
experiences, previous discrediting of the woman's sexuality, and fears
of infertility, pregnancy, sexually transmitted diseases, or fear of her
emotional and physical safety" (Basson 2002c, p. 358). As seen in this
quote, the "psychological" issues she lists could easily be interpreted as
linked to socio-political, gender-based inequalities. With that said, there
might be practical reasons for framing them in individual terms, as she
herself and her publication audiences tend to be physicians addressing
individual women's sexual complaints in a clinical setting.

Lori Brotto is another researcher who has worked within the channels
of sexual medicine, but challenges a fully medicalized view of women's
sexual problems as envisioned by the leaders of Big Pharma's sexual
revolution. Brotto has a PhD in clinical psychology from the University
of British Columbia. She later completed a post-doctoral fellowship in
Reproductive and Sexual Medicine in the same sexual medicine hospital unit as Basson. Brotto was one of the committee members tasked
to revise section on FSD in the fifth edition of the American Psychiatric Association's *Diagnostic and Statistical Manual of Mental Disorders*.
Reflecting their belief in Basson's sexual response cycle, they successfully advocated for the removal of both HSDD and FSAD from the FSD
classification, replacing them with sexual interest/arousal disorder. Her
more recent work aims at validating asexual identity through empirical
research (Brotto, Knudson, Inskip, Rhodes, & Erskine, 2010).

Brotto's work has also focused on the promise of "mindfulness-based
training" for sexual problems. Brotto (2011) defines mindfulness as "the
practice of intentionally being fully aware of one's thoughts, emotions,
and physical sensations, without judgement" (p. 215). She explains its
relevance to solving sexual problems:

Because mindfulness exerts its effects by deliberately bringing one's
full awareness to the here and now, otherwise intrusive and distracting
thoughts are left to the periphery of one's awareness, and there may be
more attunement to subtle signs of pleasure or arousal. Judgments about
one's (in)ability to become sexually excited and the fear of a partner's
rejection or disapproval float through one's conscious thoughts like clouds

bouncing across the larger landscape. Importantly, if one can describe such distractions as "just thoughts," their emotional valence is lessened. The sensation of pain may be experienced purely as a physical sensation, without the multitude of layers of affective and cognitive suffering. By learning to "ride out" the sensation of pain, the woman with dyspareunia may develop a new relationship with her pain – one that is removed of its emotional skin. (p. 216)

Mindfulness training has parallels to Masters and Johnson's recommended "sensate focus" as a treatment for (particularly men's) sexual problems, a technique that sex therapists have used widely for decades. During this kind of homework treatment, sex therapists advise couples to concentrate on touching various body parts of the body for certain periods of time, working their way up to genital touching. Understanding problems as influenced by interpersonal and contextual factors, and enhancing them with focused efforts towards sexual sensation, might be a safer and more effective way to deal with sexual problems than simply taking a pill.

The New View goes a step further, however, in challenging the very basis of sexual pharmaceuticals. It questions the discourse of sexual "function" and "dysfunction," and highlights the role of profit in motivating medicine's interest in treating sexual difficulties with a magic-bullet cure. The New View has made use of tactics inspired by women's health activism and "anti-corporate" activism to challenge the ethics of global, multinational industries such as Big Tobacco and Big Pharma (Tiefer, 2008). As a former medical-sexology-insider-turned-feminist-sex-therapist-turned-social constructionist, Leonore Tiefer, an associate clinical professor at the New York University School of Medicine, was well positioned to lead this movement. With the best combination of wit, humour, and political passion, she once bragged, "ah, the joys of being ahead of one's time!" (Tiefer, 2007, p. 473). Trained in biology and psychology, Tiefer began working as a clinical psychologist in a New York City urology department in the 1980s. As urologists began to use penile injections, implants, and vacuum pumps to treat impotence in men, she began to publish her critique of these reductionist approaches (Tiefer, 1986). She noted the social pressures for men to maintain a narrowly defined masculine sexuality based on a hard penis and a guaranteed performance, the increase references to "impotence" in the psychological literature since the 1970s, just as the term "frigidity" was finally losing currency (p. 579), and the tendency to blame "wives" or significant others when attempts to solve men's erectile difficulties failed (Tiefer, 1983). Her experience working with urologists taught her that "the field of men's sexuality was not only small but marginalized, a locus of teasing and stigma for the physicians involved" (Tiefer, 2006b, p. 285). She recognized that urologists' enthusiasm for more biological explanations of understanding men's sexual difficulties and technological means of improving erections was part of the quest for the expansion of urology's dwindling client base, legitimacy, and profits.

When Viagra was approved in 1998 and the race to find a Viagra equivalent for women was declared, Tiefer decided it was time to take direct action.[10] Against the backdrop of Goldstein's efforts to "pre-organize" (Fishman, 2004) the FSD market through a series of consensus-building conferences, she encouraged colleagues to submit papers. She wrote an article for the Boston women's newspaper, *Sojourner* (Tiefer, 1999), co-authored an op-ed for the *Los Angeles Times* (Tiefer and Tavris, 1999), and organized a seminar critiquing FSD that drew a favourable review in the *Boston Globe* (Kong, 1999). She and other concerned professionals handed out hundreds of copies of these media pieces and, as she reflects, "suddenly, we were activists" (Tiefer, 2008, p.70). Since then, Tiefer and other New View collaborators have been interviewed in almost every major news story on FSD and have published their critiques widely in academic sources (see, for example, Cacchioni & Tiefer, 2012; Kaschak & Tiefer, 2001; Loe, 2004a, 2004b, Potts & Tiefer, 2006). Filmmaker Liz Canner's (2011) documentary about the sexual pharmaceutical industry and journalist Roy Moynihan's publications in the *British Medical Journal* (2003; Moynihan & Mintzes, 2010) have offered further support for the New View's position.

Tiefer's work has been most prolific, deconstructing the frameworks and assumptions at the heart of these ploys, and calling for the return of "humanistic" models of addressing sexual problems in numerous publications (e.g., Tiefer, 2006a, 2012). She uses the term humanistic in reference to humanistic psychology and the human potential movement of the 1960s and 70s (Tiefer, 2006a). Humanistic sex therapy incorporates group treatment for couples and individuals, body imagery work, and consciousness-raising. Tiefer does not elaborate on her views of particular methods, but deems the overall goals of 'empowerment,' 'authentic communication,' and 'sensory awareness' to be more effective than a magic bullet approach to solving sexual problems.

Although humanistic sexology may belie its own social constructions, Tiefer has also embraced a social constructivist approach to her critique of the medicalization of sexual problems. She frequently references Michel Foucault (1979), Jeffrey Weeks (1991), John D'Emilio and Estelle B. Freedman (1988), and other historians who trace shifts in the historical construction of expert knowledge on sexuality. Also known for her use of metaphors, her best-known maxim, "sex is more like dancing than digestion," summarizes the crux of her views.

In 2000, with the collaboration of an interdisciplinary group of thirteen colleagues, Tiefer began to draft a manifesto on the New View of Women's Sexual Problems, and the New View Campaign was officially launched (Tiefer, 2001). Described as informed by a mélange of a social constructionsist perspective on sexual norms and ideals, psycho-social theories adopted by feminist sexual advice practitioners, and World Association of Sexology and World Health Organization decrees on "sexual rights" (Tiefer, 2002, p. 67), the manifesto was a direct challenge and a useful alternative to medicalized approaches. Its classification system has since been used to counter medicalized definitions of FSD, as an educational tool, as a means of justifying the need for feminist research on sexual enjoyment, and as a framework for sexual health practitioners.

According to the classification system, a less lucrative and more accurate way of understanding and classifying women's sexual problems would be to emphasize social factors as the most important influences on women's experiences of such problems. The New View decries the fact that socio-political factors often get "lumped into the catchall category of 'psychogenic causes'" in the medical literature on FSD (Working Group for a New View of Women's Sexual Problems, 2001, p. 4). In stark contrast to the medical model, the New View highlights a multitude of socio-political factors first and includes the most points under this category. Medical factors fall last with the fewest examples. The classification scheme is as follows.

**Sexual Problems Due to Socio-Cultural, Political, or Economic Factors**

   A. Ignorance and anxiety due to inadequate sex education, lack of access to health services, or other social constraints:
      1. Lack of vocabulary to describe subjective or physical experience
      2. Lack of information about human sexual biology and life-stage changes.

     3. Lack of information about how gender roles influence men's and women's expectations, beliefs, and behaviors.

     4. Inadequate access to information and services for contraception and abortion, STD prevention and treatment, sexual trauma, and domestic violence.

  B. Sexual Avoidance or distress due to perceived inability to meet cultural norms regarding correct or ideal sexuality, including:

     1. Anxiety or shame about one's body, sexual attractiveness, or sexual responses.

     2. Confusion or shame about one's sexual orientation or identity, or about sexual fantasies and desires.

  C. Inhibitions due to conflict between the sexual norms of one's subculture or culture of origin and those of the dominant culture.

  D. Lack of interest, fatigue, or lack of time due to family and work obligations.

I. Sexual Problems Relating to Partner and Relationship

  A. Inhibition, avoidance, or distress arising from betrayal, dislike, or fear of partner, partner's abuse or couple's unequal power, or arising from partner's negative patterns of communication.

  B. Discrepancies in desire for sexual activity, or in preferences for various sexual activities.

  C. Ignorance or inhibitions about communicating preferences or initiating, pacing, or shaping sexual activities.

  D. Loss of sexual interest and reciprocity as a result of conflicts over commonplace issues such as money, schedules, relatives, or resulting from traumatic experiences, e.g., infertility or the death of a child.

  E. Inhibitions in arousal or spontaneity due to partner's health status or sexual problems.

II. Sexual Problems Due to Psychological Factors

  A. Inhibitions in arousal or spontaneity due to:

     1. Past experiences of physical, sexual, or emotional abuse.

     2. General personality problems with attachment, rejection, co-operation, or entitlement.

     3. Depression or anxiety.

  B. Sexual inhibition due to fear of sexual acts or their possible consequences, e.g., pain during intercourse, pregnancy,

        sexually transmitted disease, loss of partner, loss of
        reputation.
IV.  Sexual Problems Due to Medical Factors

Pain or lack of physical response during sexual activity despite a supportive and safe interpersonal situation, adequate sexual knowledge,
and positive sexual attitudes. Such problems can arise from:
        A.  Numerous local or systemic medical conditions affecting
            neurological, neurovascular, circulatory, endocrine, or other
            systems of the body.
        B.  Pregnancy, sexually transmitted diseases, or other sex-related
            conditions.
        C.  Side-effects of many drugs, medications, or medical
            treatments.
        D.  Iatrogenic conditions.

## Conclusions

Drug companies are led first and foremost by the bottom line, using
increasingly commercialized strategies to sell their pills and the illness
categories they claim their magic-bullet solutions will fix. The medicalization of female sexual dysfunction, inspired by the search for a
"pink" Viagra and its potential profits, has been widely interpreted
as a classic case of pharmaceutical disease mongering. Through the
funding of clinical trials research, continuing medical education, drug
company spokespeople (along with their own clinics, websites, media
appearances, and self-help books), documentaries, and "public health"
websites, the industry is attempting to create a market of women who
self-identify as having some form of FSD and who would purchase a
drug treatment if and when one is ever approved and successfully marketed. The approval of a drug would depend primarily on the maker's
finding a way to design a trial with concrete results distinguishable
from the placebos that have so far proved to be so effective.

    The medical textbook on FSD by Goldstein et al. (2006) concludes by
stating, "[w]e look forward to the future when the biologically focused
health-care clinician has more pharmaceutical agents available with
high levels of robust evidence supporting their safe and effective use
in women with sexual health problems" (pg. 747). A decade and a half
after cries of a Big Pharma–induced sexual revolution were first heard,
however, it seems possible that such a drug will always pose problems,
whether related to efficacy, endpoints, safety, the risk-to-benefit ratio,

or simply the wider reality of the power of social influences in shaping how sexuality is understood and experienced. Each attempt to find a one-size-fits-all understanding of women's sexual dissatisfaction, particularly a physiological one, has failed. New drugs are still in the pipeline, but all those introduced so far have proved no more effective than a placebo. Women's (and men's) sexual problems are shaped by historical and contemporary socio-political and economic factors that cannot be neutralized by a drug that alters genital blood flow, hormones, or the central nervous system. As the New View argues, there is no magic-bullet cure for something as complex, varied, relational, social, mutable, and diverse as sexuality.

## 2 Treating Women's Sexual Pain: Biomedicalized, Demedicalized, and Do-It-Yourself Approaches

In the feminist critique of female sexual dysfunction (FSD), much ink has been spilled about the medicalization of dysfunctional arousal, desire, and orgasm, but much less about its fourth subset, sexual pain (American Psychiatric Association [APA], 2000, 2013). Practitioners and critics alike recognize that sexual pain has unique features compared to other sexual difficulties (Boyer, Goldfinger, Thibault-Gagnon, & Pukall, 2011; Peer Commentaries, 2005). Although desire, arousal, and orgasm lend themselves quite easily to debate as to whether they are objectively measurable phenomena relevant to the domain of health (Meana, 2010), sexual pain might have a more obvious relationship to biomedicine's expertise in pain pathways and pain reduction.

As a blockbuster sexual pharmaceutical for enhancing women's sexual desire, arousal, and orgasm remains elusive, the pharmaceutical industry and the researchers they fund increasingly turn their attention to developing drugs for sexual pain. A breadth of medical terms, classifications, and treatments now surrounds women's genital and sexual pain. Health professionals use pharmacological solutions to sexual pain, but significantly, most advocate patient-centred desensitization therapies as most effective for its management. These techniques usually are taught and administered by health care practitioners whose services can be difficult to access and unaffordable. And yet it seems women could engage in these decidedly low-tech therapies without the help of an expert.

One-third of the women I interviewed experienced sexual pain of some kind, so it is important to explore sexual pain and its treatment in further detail. In this chapter I unpack biomedical and other ways of understanding and treating sexual pain. I examine sexual pain pharmaceuticals, professionally led desensitization techniques, and do-it-yourself, inexpensive approaches to treating sexual pain that have been adopted at the grassroots level. I draw on expert literature that describes the more biomedical approaches, as well as my own field-work examining professionally guided, but low-tech, desensitization techniques seldom discussed in published literature, but commonly used by sexual medicine clinicians and pelvic physiotherapists to treat sexual pain. Comparing these approaches highlights the connections between medicalized, biomedicalized, demedicalized, and grassroots approaches. I also suggest that barriers to access and lack of affordability might inhibit the widespread uptake of biomedical or professionally led methods.

Most salient to the central themes of this book, however, this chapter demonstrates the limited view of sexuality that informs the desired endpoints of these treatments – and of treatments for sexual problems more generally. The restoration of penis-vagina penetration is the unequivocal goal of all sexual pain therapies I have read about, heard described in interviews with sex experts and lay women, and observed in pelvic physiotherapy sessions. Reaching this goal is not necessarily linked to enhanced sexual pleasure. It does not necessarily disrupt the power relations of heterosex, the narrow terms in which "real," "successful," or "good" heterosex is judged, or the importance sex is afforded. Thus, no matter how educational or empowering individual women perceive some of the more patient-centred exercises to be, they are based on an individualized framework of understanding sexuality. As I discuss later in the book, this framework is based on the assumption that heteronormative sexual ideals are necessarily goals to be worked upon, even when they are not pleasurable and cause distress.

## Defining Sexual Pain

In this chapter, and throughout this book, I use "sexual pain" with the understanding that this is a contested term with myriad origins. The type of sexual pain that is medicalized is not infrequent pain with intercourse or pain caused by particularly rough or violent sex; rather, it is typically associated with chronic genital pain and/or the thinning of vaginal tissue during menopause. As I have examined with Janine Farrell (Farrell & Cacchioni, 2012), historically, although the medical profession documented pain and itching in and around women's genitals (Friedrich, 1987), it deemed these sensations to be psychosomatic or "in a woman's head" (Grace, 2000; McKay, 1989).[1] In response to such assertions, grassroots patient advocacy groups such as the National Vulvodynia Association (NVA) have fought for medicalization to further and improve access to medical resources.

In the realm of contemporary sexual medicine, the American Psychiatric Association's *Diagnostic and Statistical Manual of Mental Disorders* (DSM) has been granted the most legitimacy for defining sexual pain. The fourth edition of the DSM, known as DSM-IV-TR (APA, 2000), classifies "sexual pain disorders" as a subset of FSD, dividing the category into "dyspareunia," defined as "recurrent or persistent genital pain associated with sexual intercourse" that causes significant "distress and/or interpersonal difficulty," and "vaginismus," "a recurrent or persistent involuntary spasm of the musculature of the outer third of the vagina that interferes with intercourse."[2] As chronic genital pain is increasingly understood as a form of chronic pain like any other, however, there is a movement to declassify it as a sexual dysfunction and reclassify it as chronic pain syndrome (Binik, 2005), as the International Society for the Study of Vulvar Disease already does. While these debates continue (see Peer Commentaries, 2005, for details), the majority of health professionals involved in the treatment of sexual pain – including former sex therapist Leonore Tiefer – agree that the medicalization of sexual pain facilitates "clinical inquiry and treatment, professional education, health insurance coverage, and research attention" (Tiefer, 2005, p. 50). In a rare published comment on sexual pain, Tiefer claims that, "as long as there are expert-based listings of sexual dysfunctions, we do women a disservice by failing to include pain as one of them," adding a caveat that she would be "happy to dispense with such norms entirely" (p. 51).

When I began my research into chronic sexual pain, I harboured the common perception that ongoing sexual pain problems likely stemmed from past experiences of trauma – for example, a history of sexual abuse. Yet, at a sexual pain workshop in Vancouver, several attendees who identified as having chronic sexual pain claimed that their greatest relief was finding practitioners who understood their condition as *unrelated* to a history of sexual abuse. One participant made a point of seeking me out to tell me, "I want to be clear that these pain disorders do not stem from sexual abuse." Another took me aside to state, "For your study it's important to realize that we have to debunk this sexual abuse myth or else it makes it impossible for women to get proper treatment." The sexual medicine specialist I interviewed similarly lamented,

"[Non-sexual medicine physicians] will insist ... I got this referral the other day that I'll show you from a gynecologist. She *insisted* the patient had been abused but was not admitting it." Based on her research and clinical experience, this specialist strongly disagreed with such a characterization. In addition, among the eleven women I interviewed who identified as having some form of chronic genital pain leading to sexual pain, all but one claimed either no history of sexual abuse or no history predating the sensation of chronic genital pain. Like the women at the workshop, they expressed their frustration at this commonplace misunderstanding, which they perceived as having prevented them from receiving adequate pain management.

Most biomedical research on women's sexual pain explains chronic genital pain in relation to the immune system, skin hypersensitivity, allergies, chronic nerve pain and congestion, and imbalanced hormones and neurotransmitters (Farrell & Cacchioni, 2012). For instance, as one explanation, the sexual medicine specialist I interviewed used a neurological "conversational" metaphor and imagery depicting the body's "inner message system." She stated, "We know there is kind of crisscross talk between the immune cells in the blood stream and the nerve endings ... generating this ongoing pain." She elaborated:

> White blood cells release their chemicals and when they do, there's inflammation that sensitizes the nerve endings [which] send more pain signals up the spinal cord up to the brain, and when the nerve endings, sensory nerve endings are overactive, the nerve cell body in the spinal cord becomes chemically changed and sends the message the opposite way. We used to think sensory nerves just sent a message from the periphery up to the brain, but we [now] know sensory nerves also send messages the other way from the cell body in the spinal cord to the skin nerve ending. So when they get overreactive that way, they also get overreactive this way. The cells are themselves releasing chemicals, and guess what the chemicals do from the nerve endings? They attract white blood cells. So, it's this whole cycle. It's this cycle going on and on.

Similarly, the pelvic physiotherapist who led the workshop I attended used an "alarm bell" metaphor to explain the neurological components of chronic genital pain. After attending the workshop, I noted in my fieldwork diary: "She drew a diagram of the brain and the spinal cord. She explained that when pain stemming from, say, an abrasion goes untreated, neurotransmitters in the spinal cord turn up their 'alarm system.' So then when the area is touched at all, 'danger receptor alarms go off'." These discourses parallel other discourses on immunity. According to Martin (1994), immunity was once described in terms of "stress" compromising the body's defences, but it is now described as a system that can be "tuned up" to fight against the body's environment. Under this logic, drugs treating chronic genital pain are designed to "fight" or "reverse" the "pain cycle."

A growing body of feminist qualitative research, like my own, explicitly emphasizes the role of social factors in shaping women's experiences of sexual pain (rather than focusing on the root cause). For example, Ayling and Ussher (2008), Grace and MacBride-Stewart (2007), Kaler (2006), and Marriott and Thompson (2008) use empirical qualitative methods (primarily interviews) to examine women's experiences and understandings of sexual pain. According to these interviews, chronic genital pain is seen as most distressing in the context of hegemonic understandings of intercourse as the only "real" heterosex. Similar to the findings that I discuss in the following chapter, the women in their research most commonly experienced compulsory heterosexuality as an imperative to have penetrative penis-vagina sex with a male partner, a practice they felt was integral to the longevity of their relationships and their identities as heterosexual women.

## Treating Sexual Pain: Biomedical Approaches

As I have argued with Janine Farrell (Farrell & Cacchioni, 2012), professionals who specialize in treating sexual pain tend to agree that multifactorial, multidisciplinary approaches to treatment are necessary for this extremely complex, heterogeneous problem (Boyer et al., 2011; Graziottin & Brotto, 2004; Landry, Bergeron, Dupuis, & Desrochers, 2008). A chapter on sexual pain in a definitive textbook on "sexual dysfunctions" (Payne, Bergeron, Khalifé, & Binik, 2006) explains that medical interventions for sexual pain "lie on a continuum from relatively minor to invasive methods, operating largely on a trial and error basis" and with little empirical support. Depending on the type of sexual pain, medical treatment may begin with "[l]ocal topical treatments (such as sitz baths), progressing to topical medical treatments involving corticosteroid, estrogen, or lidocaine cream, to oral medications such as calcium citrate, corticosteroids, or fluconazole. Should such methods fail, progressively more invasive approaches are recommended, such as interferon injections, neurophysiologic treatments, and finally surgical excision via vestibuloplasty, or partial to total vestibulectomy" (p. 474). Vestibulectomy is described as a "minor surgical process, which consists of the excision of the hymen and sensitive areas of the vestibule." Healing takes up to eight weeks and the "success" rate has been estimated between 43 and 100 per cent. "Success" is defined as the minimizing or complete reduction of pain during intercourse.

Although the desensitization techniques I describe later in the chapter remain the cornerstone of treatment, biomedical treatments for sexual pain increasingly are proposed. The intravaginal injection of Botox, the trade name of the highly poisonous substance botulinum toxin, has been under consideration as a treatment for vaginismus for the past ten years, but each study conducted so far has involved a sample of only sixty or fewer women (Ghazizadeh and Nikzad, 2004; Pacik, 2009; Shafik & Eli-Sibai, 2000). On 11 August 2010, the US Food and Drug Administration (FDA) approved clinical trials of Botox to treat vaginismus. The trial involves injecting 150 units of Botox intravaginally in thirty patients under general anesthetic, followed by dilation therapy, wherein tapered, wax-candle-like dilators (invented by Masters and Johnson) – or vaginal accommodators, as they are sometimes called – of graduated widths are inserted over time.

Peter P. Pacik, the principal investigator of the FDA clinical trials, is a cosmetic surgeon with his own "surgicenter" in Manchester, New Hampshire. By the time Pacik began conducting clinical trials, he claimed to have treated twenty patients in his practice with off-label Botox at a 90 per cent "success" rate. Of these patients, Pacik reported sixteen were able to achieve intercourse in two to three weeks, three advanced to the fifth or sixth of six dilators, and one was "unable to advance beyond the smallest dilator" and was therefore "considered a failure" (Pacik, 2009, p. 455–6).

Pacik's emphasis on the role of Botox in his treatment, however, must be considered carefully. In all the hype surrounding Botox for vaginismus, the significance of the dilation stage of the process has been downplayed. As I learned when I called his office and spoke to the receptionist, a key part of this treatment is the insertion of a penis-sized dilator while the patient is still under local anesthetic, immediately post-injection. The patient is then encouraged to slip the dilator in and out several times over the course of the next hour. When the patient is discharged from the surgical centre, she is asked to keep a "size 4 out of 6" dilator inside her vagina for twenty-four hours. The following day, when the anesthesia has worn off, she is to return to what Pacik's assistant termed "dilator boot camp," or one to two days of assisted dilation. It then takes months of self-administered dilation for the patient to achieve pain-free sexual intercourse. In other words, the effect of Botox is the temporary relaxation of the muscles. Along with a local anesthetic, Botox simply speeds up the pace at which the woman can progress in dilation. Dilation, which I describe in more detail later in this chapter, is an older, low-tech, inexpensive approach to treating vaginismus, and can be done without professional guidance. As his receptionist explained, Pacik's treatment package costs US$5,400, including the in-house procedure, "dilation boot camp," and counselling on how to use dilators at home.

What sets Botox apart from previous generations of drugs to manage sexual pain is the way it was marketed to the public even before its approval for this use. Pacik and his co-author Joni Cole have been advertising Botox as a treatment for vaginismus through a book directed towards lay audiences entitled *When Sex Seems Impossible* (2010). In it, they label all other clinically supported treatment techniques dealing with vaginismus as "conservative," in the sense of their failure to adopt new technologies. Pacik uses regulatory loopholes on marketing drugs not approved for a given use by other clever means as well. For instance, he has released a YouTube video exhorting women who have tried the procedure off-label to share their success stories online through blogs and websites. With the results of his trials imminent, an article in the November 2011 edition of *Cosmopolitan* magazine featured an editorial describing one of his patients' "success" stories. Yet, in a paper for a clinical audience, Pacik tempered his claims, concluding that ongoing, multidisciplinary "support after treatment is critical" (Pacik, 2011, p. 1163).

Of his career trajectory from reconstructive surgeon to cosmetic plastic surgeon to self-proclaimed innovator in the treatment of vaginismus, Pacik reflects, "[t]here comes a time in every person's life that routine 12–18 hour work days must come to an end. I made this decision in the mid 1980s to begin concentrating on the field of cosmetic surgery."[3] Elsewhere he explains, "In 2005, a patient called the office to ask if I would treat her vaginismus with Botox. I never heard the term nor did I learn anything about this condition in medical school. I was stunned by the lack of medical information. I had enough experience with Botox that I was confident I could help her. The outcome was successful and my patient was finally able to achieve pain free intercourse … As I treated more women, I realized that the treatment of vaginismus became a 'calling'."[4]

In 2012 a non-medicated cosmetic branded as Neogyn Vulvar Soothing Cream was released with the endorsement of some members of the International Society for the Study of Women's Sexual Health. The active ingredient of the cream is cutaneous lysate – cell culture vessels that are harvested, washed, and prepared for "cell disruption." These are "obtained from a biotechnology derived process following stringent manufacturing procedures from a dedicated cell bank" in Switzerland.[5] In a press release by the company, Andrew Goldstein, the same doctor who promotes Lybrido and Lybridos, is quoted as making the following rather vague statement: "For years, I've had patients suffer from vulvodynia, yet vulvar pain is commonly misdiagnosed or under reported, as many women are reluctant to talk about their symptoms … Neogyn Vulvar Soothing Cream may give women coping with vulvar pain a soothing option; and it can be used in conjunction with other vulvodynia treatments" (para. 3). Vulvodynia refers to pain and itching in and around the genitals with or without sexual or other contact (McKay, 1989).

Then, in March 2013, with very little media fanfare in the lead-up to its FDA approval, a drug called Osphena was approved for the treatment of menopausal-related sexual pain. Although the drug works using an entirely different mechanism than Viagra and is approved for use in a very select population, once again the popular press chimed, "Pharma's race for a 'pink Viagra' finally has a winner, and the promises for it are grand" (Block, 2013, para. 1). Osphena is a selective estrogen-receptor modulator that mimics estrogen and allegedly treats symptoms of "vulvo-vaginal atrophy," the thinning of vaginal tissue caused by a reduction in estrogen levels (Portman, Bachmann, & Simon, 2013). As Block (2013) notes, the rate and severity of this diagnosis are controversial, as most menopausal women will experience it to some degree as a "normal" part of aging. The "statistically significant improvement" with use of Osphena reported by the company is based on two twelve-week studies funded by Shionogi and QuatRx, the drug's developers. The subjects of the studies were women who self-reported their "most bothersome symptom" (MBS) as "vulvo-vaginal dryness." Over the course of 12 weeks, 806 and then 605 women taking the drug experienced an improvement of less than 0.5 per cent in MBS compared with women taking a placebo (Block, 2013, para. 23). Moreover, clinical trials revealed side effects and risks including, but not limited to, blood clots, urinary tract infections, cancer, stroke, increased instances of hot flashes, and yeast infections (para. 21). Due to Osphena's similarity to estrogen, critics have also expressed concern over potential off-label prescription use as a form of menopausal hormone replacement therapy without adequate testing.

## Desensitization Techniques: A Demedicalized Approach

Despite all these highly technological developments, many sexual pain experts continue to advocate for the least-invasive approaches with the fewest side effects. The health care practitioners I interviewed and those described by women in my study seemed to advocate what Carol Wolkowitz and I have termed "body work" approaches to desensitizing women's sexual pain (Cacchioni & Wolkowitz, 2011; see also Twigg, Cohen, Nettleton, & Wolkowitz, 2011).[6] In Vancouver, all of the practitioners who offered these services were women; indeed, in North America, it seems to be mainly women who perform these treatments, although there are some exceptions in the medical field. For example, Andrew Goldstein and his colleague Dr Stanley Marinoff are well known for performing desensitization therapies at the Centers for Vulvovaginal Disorders in Washington, DC, New York City, and Annapolis, Maryland.[7]

Desensitization techniques emphasizing cognitive behavioural patterns, relaxation, and other "mind-body" connections are considered the most proven strategies for the treatment of sexual pain (Payne et al., 2006). These methods can be seen as demedicalized in that they reach beyond conventional medical techniques and emphasize "mind" and "body," but were born out of pragmatic needs, rather than an explicit "anti-medicalization" project (Tiefer, 2012). They are not entirely nonmedicalized, as they involve expert authority, some very basic technologies, and money. The sexual medicine specialist and the pelvic physiotherapists I interviewed and observed in this study claimed that professionals in their field adopted these methods through commonsense thinking about how to help their patients, largely because drugs alone were not proven to be useful in the long term. In addition to prescribing pain medication, sexual medicine physicians help patients gradually get used to the sensation of having physical (and eventually sexual) genital contact (Basson, Wierman, van Lankveld, & Brotto, 2010).

As is standard in a gynecological procedure of any kind, providers of these treatments employ various techniques to make sure their patients or clients are comfortable and to establish an "objective" medical environment. When I observed rounds in sexual medicine, an entire session was dedicated to addressing legal challenges, embarrassment, physical discomfort, and other issues arising from diagnostic exams performed by men and women doctors or desensitization techniques performed by women physicians. During this meeting, the team of doctors developed protocols for establishing boundaries while touching women intimately. These included draping techniques, using verbal signals to alert the woman to what they would be doing, and offering the woman the option of having a chaperone. They also discussed what to do if "a patient becomes involuntarily aroused during the clinical process." One doctor suggested, "Move away, stop, and have a face-to-face discussion about it." These kinds of measures reflect the findings of Emerson (1970a, 1970b) over four decades ago – mainly, that health practitioners who touch a woman's vulva must negotiate the contradiction between the medical view of the vulva as a body part like any other and the idea that this body part must be approached with extreme care.

Desensitization body work treatments use a slow, gradual approach to treating sexual pain, emphasizing the patient's active participation in clinical procedures and sexual activities. Describing these techniques, the sexual medicine specialist I interviewed explained, "We'll wait until she's done a little bit more self-touch before we actually attempt to see what's actually going on in the vagina." She also might prescribe pre-exam exercises, including "kegal exercises, relaxation techniques, and bearing down techniques" that enhance the woman's capacity to control her vagina. (A kegal exercise consists of contracting and relaxing one's pelvic floor muscles.) The in-house exam itself is designed with "therapeutic" as well as diagnostic intentions. As the specialist explained, "It's not conducted like a routine such as a Pap smear. It's done much more slowly," with the woman actively participating in the process. While the patient sits up holding a mirror, the physician explains the functions of various parts of the vagina and then leads her through variations on a kegal exercise. The physician I interviewed explained the rationale for this approach:

> She's feeling like, you know, 'I'm not just having this done to me.' You know it's not enough to tell her that she can tell me when to stop anytime. It's a lot easier if she's right there and to have her help as much as possible. Her spreading the labia is much better, for one, it's much easier, you've still got two hands left! And number two, you know, that's permission for you to go ahead. I mean, there's nothing clearer than her saying, 'Okay, take a

look.' It means she's doing. She's helping. And they are much rougher on themselves than I am.

Once the patient is comfortable with being touched by the doctor or touching herself, the doctor asks her to "tighten and withdraw," doing a range of kegal and reverse kegal exercises so the patient can see that "Oh, my goodness, I can control this." A reverse kegal exercise consists of relaxing one's pelvic floor beyond what one perceives to be a neutral state, and involves a slight pushing motion. The patient is then asked to insert her own finger into her vulva or to insert the doctor's finger, whichever she is more comfortable with. Even so, as the sexual medicine doctor explained, "some of them get quite faint if they have never been looked at or touched before, even if you're going very gently and very slowly, in tiny steps. She may become very dizzy, so you want to get her down [on a couch] quickly." Once she seems ready to attempt penetration, she is prescribed vaginal dilators, and is encouraged to spend time with these devices at home, graduating to a full-sized, penis-shaped dildo, and then to "the real thing."

Treatment by pelvic physiotherapists encourages women to become aware of their pain triggers (diet, movement, times during a menstrual cycle, sexual activity); to understand exactly where they feel pain; to learn how to strengthen the pelvic floor muscle; to learn how to relax the pelvic floor muscles; and, finally, to recognize when these muscles are tense or relaxed. Practitioners explain that all of these lessons are tricky since, according to them, women in general "aren't aware of that part of their anatomy" and rarely discuss how it should feel "normally." For example, some women with genital pain think that sexual intercourse, or simply inserting a tampon, is supposed to be somewhat painful. To test muscle function, the pelvic physiotherapist asks the patient to do a kegal while she inserts a finger into the vulva and/or anus. She then asks the patient to contract and release. In cases where the patient with vulvar pain is extremely anxious, the therapist might use Xylocaine, a numbing gel, to desensitize her.

The next step is biofeedback, a method used to raise the patient's awareness of, and ability to relax, an injured body part. The technique involves connecting the body part to a computer using a sensory device, allowing the patient to visualize its movements. In a simple line graph, the computer screen displays the tensing and relaxing of the body part, which helps the patient understand what "tensed" or "relaxed" feels like in an area where tension has become so normalized that she does not recognize it. The readout displays a flat line when muscles are relaxed, sharp peaks and valleys when they are not. In pelvic physiotherapy, the vagina is connected to the biofeedback machine either with electrodes placed on the thigh and anus or with a sensory device inserted into the vagina. Movements are guided by specific exercises such as kegal and reverse kegal. In more advanced sessions with a patient who is near the end of her treatment, the physiotherapist will ask her to create different kinds of lines on the biofeedback screen by tensing or relaxing her pelvic floor muscles in different ways. The therapist will ask the patient to do a series of "ramps," "spikes," "gentle releases," and "releases" for about twenty minutes.

Figure 2.1. Biofeedback Readout

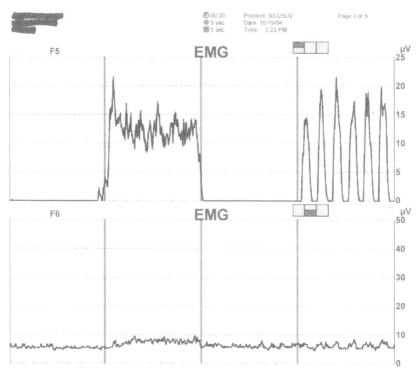

Note: Used in pelvic physiotherapy to measure when pelvic floor muscles are "tight" or "relaxed." Sharp peaks represent tightness and dips and valleys represent relaxed. Source: Anonymous.

Another physiotherapy method is pelvic massage, although there is debate among the pelvic physiotherapists I interviewed about its effectiveness. One physiotherapist would massage the pelvic floor muscles both internally and externally to "loosen" the area and soften and stretch the tissue. Pelvic massage also incorporates "trigger point work" – in that physiotherapist's words, touching the vagina "below the pain threshold." In her opinion, this eases the process of penile-vaginal penetration and desensitizes painful areas. As she explained, "you're working with the muscles, you're making sure that they're lengthened, that they're not in spasm, they are able to relax, that they can get stronger. But you're also dealing with very reactive muscles so that when you touch them, they can go like this [making a fist]."

## Making Sense of Desensitization Techniques

The women I interviewed who had accessed professionally led desensitization techniques talked about them as effective in reducing pain and achieving the goal of less painful and sometimes pain-free intercourse. Highlighting a key point in what might undermine the power of medicalization, however, they perceived these treatments as difficult to access and unaffordable in the long term.

The women in this study who eventually were referred to the sexual medicine unit and/or pelvic physiotherapy said they were pleased by the careful attention their bodies received during these desensitization sessions. Generally, they claimed to like the "hands-on" attention, because they felt an "expert" was taking their bodily complaints seriously. The majority claimed to have previously encountered general practitioners or non-sexual medicine gynecologists who either "ignored" or "dismissed" their physical concerns or, in some cases, failed to approach their bodies carefully. The story of Courtney, a twenty-five-year-old student who identified as having vaginismus, illustrates this point. Like many women with an intense fear of penetration, Courtney was referred to a non-sexual medicine gynecologist who failed miserably at the task of approaching her body. He first promised her that "he just wanted to look and see," but "he just started poking away … and eventually tried to put his finger inside." Courtney "screamed" because "it was so horrible and painful." The gynecologist responded to her lack of compliance by saying, "You know, if you can't let me do this, then I can't help you." He advised her to try using "birthday candles" or "a carrot" to retrain her body. Courtney contrasted this to the careful approach taken to touching her body when she was treated at the sexual medicine unit of the hospital. There, the sexual medicine specialist "made it really clear that I didn't *have* to do anything. We'll do it at your own pace." Ironically, when her sexual medicine physician prescribed vaginal dilators, she saw this in positive terms, even though dilators are not very different from wax candles in size or shape.

Although a visual ethic of avoidance characterizes traditional pelvic exams through careful draping techniques and the patient's inability to view the examination process (Heath, 1986; Henslin & Biggs, 1971), a visual ethic of looking is part and parcel of the development of desensitization techniques. Women have been encouraged to look at their vulvas as a way to reappropriate the male medical gaze since the early days of the women's health movement (Davis, 2007), but "self-spectatorship is virtually unaccounted for in the traditional gynecological theatre" (Kapsalis, 1997, p. 166). It seems, however, that practitioners who specialize in treating women's sexual pain have caught on to the power of active spectatorship as a way to enhance women's sense of capacity for control, comfort, and, perhaps, enjoyment. Linda, a twenty-two-year-old pre-med student, noted, "I used to think I peed out of my clitoris … So, definitely the mirror was an amazing teaching tool for her to teach me what was going on." Another of the interviewees, Charlene, agreed, reflecting that "Most women have never even looked down there, so they don't know what they're supposed to be looking at." These comments reflect Tiefer's (1995) belief that education about sexual anatomy is one of the best forms of sex therapy.

Women in the study also prized the visual-physical feedback loop displayed on the biofeedback computer screen. Participants explained how it helped them interpret their bodily sensations. As Mika stated, "it was helpful because it was very educational how much your muscles will tense up as a result of painful sex or actual pain … You could see the activity of the muscles, the tone of your muscles, so if they were tight, you could see that on the screen and then see when you're relaxing them." Similarly, Sophie claimed that "[the biofeedback] meant that I have much greater awareness of what relaxed feels like. And it doesn't feel like being relaxed. It feels kind of like pushing. And I wasn't aware of that before. It means that I can consciously relax. I think that all of that has to do with building control."

Praise aside, the women I interviewed described also these techniques as inaccessible and/or costly. In British Columbia, sexual medicine services are covered by the provincial health care system, but waiting lists are long (four to eighteen months), and once in the system, the patient is able to access only a limited number of treatment sessions (typically four to six). Of her waiting time of six months to access these services, Mika, a twenty-two-year-old student working in retail, stated, "I felt hopeless." Danielle, a forty-four-year-old teacher, described her being on the waiting list for eighteen months as a "horrendous" and "terrible" experience. Symbolic of the heteronormative framework in which FSD, including sexual pain, is conceptualized, single women felt that their concern over their sexual pain was not taken seriously and they were often denied priority on waiting lists.

British Columbia's universal health insurance covers pelvic physiotherapy only if it is accompanied by urinary incontinence; otherwise, the therapy is available to anyone for an average price of $150 per session. There is no set number of treatments that pelvic physiotherapists recommend. The women in my study who accessed this resource had an average of five sessions, but deemed it unaffordable in the long term. Susan, a retired lab technician, saw a private pelvic physiotherapist before being referred to the one pelvic physiotherapist covered under the provincial health insurance scheme because she had the required incontinence diagnosis. Of the practitioner in private practice, she reported, "Money is quite important to her." Mika termed her pelvic physiotherapist "the most fantastic and hope-inducing out of anybody," but she was unable to "continue to keep paying the $75 per session fees" – and even that was a lower charge she was able to negotiate on a sliding scale. Her "biggest beef" was "just the fact that I feel you have to be rich to get control of this issue." Charlene, a groundstaff employee at the airport, stated that her pelvic physiotherapist's fee "was outrageous." She pointed out that, in France, similar services are covered by the national health insurance, stating, "They're so progressive. I should be there." Charlene was frustrated that the management of sexual pain was given a lower priority than "getting your tubes tied," crying, "but I have PAIN!"

**Treating Sexual Pain: Grassroots, Do-It-Yourself Options**

Given the cost, relative inaccessibility, and relatively low skill level involved in some of the desensitization techniques I described above, I wondered what resources were available at the grassroots level. In some cases, health professionals endorse a self-help approach. The health professionals I interviewed were adamant that the "homework" they set for women and their partners to do at home was equally, if not more, important than the exercises performed in their clinics. To that end, Canadian physiotherapists and gynecologists partnered to open "Come As You Are," a cooperative offering high-quality, "user-friendly" dilators online and in stores.[8] As an example of a more commercialized approach, Amy Stein, a well-known pelvic physiotherapist and author of the self-published book, *Heal Pelvic Pain* (2009) and accompanying website,[9] is a self-help guru who has appeared on numerous medical segments of popular news programs. Stein's self-help materials offer a step-by-step guide to exercises and techniques women can practise at home. But these resources also serve as an advertisement for her private New York clinic for those who want to go "beyond the basics." (Beyond Basics Physical Therapy, 2011).[10]

A notably less medicalized and less commercial forum for the do-it-yourself approach to dealing with sexual pain was the Vaginismus Awareness website.[11] Since vaginismus is commonly linked to chronic genital pain more generally, the website appealed to a wide range of women with sexual pain issues. While the anonymous author of the explicitly not-for-profit website acknowledged that "some women may really benefit from the help of a professional," she lamented the perceived need for expert guidance, and the "invisibility in the literature of the women who have actually-self treated ... on their own despite clear evidence they exist and in great numbers." She highlighted the explosion of the "growth of medical authority so that only doctors are allowed to talk about vaginismus." Finally, she offered support and suggestions for alternative modes of intimacy for women who do not wish to work towards pain free penetrative sex with step-by-step guidance on desensitization and dilation techniques for those who do. In her view, learning these techniques at home, with (or without) a partner, can be the most affordable, self-empowering approach to healing. She admitted this takes skill, but "professional, not necessarily." The website was brimming with positive reviews by women who had "self-treated." Without this site, or something like it, it seems there is an unmet need for women seeking information on self-treatment.

Although none of the women in my study mentioned the above sources, they spoke of the value of Internet information and self-help books such as *A Woman's Guide to Fear and Pain* by Goodwin and Agronin (1997), *Private Pain: It's About Life, Not Just Sex* by Katz and Tabisel (2002). These books provide detailed information about anatomy, pain triggers, and pain management, as well as sexual advice. The women in my study also accessed grassroots sexual pain support groups in the wider Vancouver community.

In feminist discussions of grassroots health movements, it is often assumed that, through grassroots support groups, "women are able to withdraw themselves from medicalization and present an opposing force" (Bransen, 1992, p. 99). Recent sociological literature, however, has attempted to unpack the presumed existence of lay knowledge untainted by "expert" knowledge. For example, in an article titled "How Lay Are Lay Beliefs?" Shaw (2002) problematizes the concept of "lay beliefs" given that "commonsense" perspectives are often "themselves based upon understandings within expert paradigms" (p. 287). It seems that, in the contemporary Information or Digital Age, the distinction between "lay" and "expert" is particularly difficult to untangle. Ironically, although desensitization techniques seemed doable on one's own with proper instructions, the support groups for sexual pain described by the women in my study seemed to be dedicated largely to "talking about different [medical] treatments" (meaning drugs), "anything that's helped you in the past or now." Mika explained that the benefit of support groups was their ability to foster a feeling of being "in control" of access to medical information. As she stated, "To be able to go to my doctor and say, 'This is what I've heard about lately. What about this?' and all this stuff" helped her "to take a more active stance on it." Group members also found it helpful to hear fellow members' opinions of pharmacological drugs. As Charlene stated, "it's good to hear both sides" before trying any medication. One participant mentioned that she had attempted a treatment known as "the Lidocaine and cotton ball treatment" after hearing about it from the group.

## Conclusions

Although the feminist critique of FSD has centred on the search for a sexual pharmaceutical aimed at enhancing women's sexual desire, arousal, and orgasm, much less has been said about the health care and pharmaceutical industry's approach to assisting women with sexual pain. Sexual pain has been medicalized through medical classification and treatment, and biomedicalized through increasingly technological treatment methods. Newly developed biomedical therapies differ from their predecessors in their cost, level of invasiveness, and degree of marketing. Alongside these trends has been the simultaneous demedicalization of sexual pain treatment through remarkably low-tech, desensitization techniques. Technically speaking, it is possible for lay women to try these techniques themselves without direct professional guidance, although they are only rarely promoted by professionals as such.

As Carol Wolkowitz and I have discussed (Cacchioni & Wolkowitz, 2011), sexual medicine specialists and pelvic physiotherapists attend to women's immediate complaints of sexual discomfort or displeasure through procedures that encourage women to feel "in control" during the procedure itself and then in sexual interactions. Their clients and patients might present with a number of physiological complaints, but their treatments are based primarily on the simple principle of enhancing women's connections to and control over their vagina. Participants who were able to access specialist sexual therapy desensitization procedures described these techniques as therapeutic and empowering. For instance, they said they found that the visualization techniques practitioners adopted helped them to connect to their bodies, rather than feeling that the techniques objectified them. Moreover, the treatments administered by practitioners offering hands-on care were highly prized for the careful, gradual, approach that encouraged women to be active participants in the overall process.

These practitioners' approaches arguably accord with feminist thinking in important ways. The therapies described in this chapter accomplish some of the objectives of 1970s consciousness-raising efforts aimed at encouraging women to "get in touch with themselves" (Davis, 2007), and parallel the emphasis on women's ability to pleasure themselves seen in the current explosion of feminist sex shops. It is not simply that desensitization procedures encourage women to overcome sexual shame, anxiety, and discomfort quite literally by facing their vulva. It is also that they see the vagina as an active organ, rather than as a passive receptacle.

Compared to a strictly pharmaceutical approach to treating women's sexual pain, a magic-bullet cure, even if it were a possibility, might not replace hands-on interactions, visual techniques, and the value women attach to them. For the most part, these therapies are seen as helping women with the privilege of access to such resources to understand and accept the ways in which their vulva/vagina looks, feels, and functions. The pharmaceutical approach to treating women's sexual difficulties, in contrast, leaves out key steps in what seems a highly tactile process that involves the therapeutic power of embodied touch and empowered looking.

Women guiding women through these exercises might be interpreted as "queering" the heteronormative script against which sexual problems are judged, as I discuss later in the book. But the very notion of queering is meant to destabilize hegemonic categorizations. Just as Haraway (1999) saw the 1970s women's self-help movement as empowering individual middle-class women without transforming wider institutions of health care or heterosex, today's practitioners operate largely within current conventions of both these institutions. Particularly with the availability of online information on do-it-yourself techniques, there seems to be no reason the majority of these low-tech techniques should require the guidance of a medical or professional expert. Moreover, whatever the approach, most treatments are measured by the restoration of penetrative sex, even though women might wish to restore other pain-free sexual activity, such as manual and oral stimulation. Insofar as the primary goal of these treatments is to allow women to participate in penetrative intercourse, they do not challenge either the heteronormative framework of "real" sex (Jackson and Scott, 2001) or the notion that we must all be sexual. They seem to enhance women's "sense" of control over (in these cases hetero) sex, but one cannot assume that sense necessarily will translate into heterosexual encounters.

Finally, as I demonstrate in the rest of the book, even if these treatments are seen as effective in making intercourse less painful, they do not seem to mediate between the often harsh way the women in my study tended to view themselves, and their partners often perceived them, simply because they are uninterested in performing, or unwilling, unable, or find it difficult to perform, the hallowed act of heterosexual intercourse.

# 3 The Limits of Normative Heterosex

Heterosexuality is far from a homogeneous identity category or set of practices, and is shaped by intersecting aspects of identity such as race, ethnicity, nationality, age, and social class. I therefore expected a fair degree of nuance, disagreement, and competing stories of navigating heterosex from the women in my study when they described their perceived sexual difficulties. There were striking similarities, however, in participants' accounts of what constitutes normative sex and the centrality of heterosexual norms for their personal, interpersonal, and social lives. All the women I interviewed shared a conscious awareness of the heteronormative script as limiting, an insight they seemed to acquire at great cost over the course of their life cycle.

Participants' overall awareness of the pressures of normative sex made sense to me, however, when I considered that their experiences were connected by three main factors. First, the vast majority identified as heterosexual; second, all had been in heterosexual relationships at some point in their lives; third, all of them did not, could not, or did not want to mirror the expectations of normative heterosex. In varying combinations, they did not desire sexual activity frequently, had difficulty with arousal, found intercourse painful, and/or could not orgasm easily or at all. These factors in and of themselves could have given rise to a distinct outlook on sex, one that would include an intense and conscious awareness of normative sexual standards, the value that is afforded to them, and in many cases, their coercive power.

In this chapter, I explore the ways in which the women in my study understood and experienced (for the most part normative hetero) sex. Most of these women embodied the contradictions of the supposed "post-feminist" age in that they were disappointed in and even traumatized by many aspects of heterosex, and yet felt immense pressure from several sources to be actively, frequently, and orgasmically heterosexual. In their shame about their primarily heterosexual shortcomings, they avoided discussing these issues with friends, a finding paralleled in Loe's (2004b) research on men's sexual difficulties. The women in my study internalized their partners' negative reactions to their sexual problems, while simultaneously expressing anger and outrage at the pressures they faced. All of this is crucial information for appreciating the "labour of love," the interpersonal sex work in which these women engage.

## Empirical Research on Sexual Freedom and the Sexual Double Standard

A growing body of empirical literature warns against what McRobbie (2006) has termed the "postfeminist masquerade" of sexual freedom. As Renold & Ringrose (2008) state, mainstream neoliberal media inundate us with representations of women as "unambiguous success stories of late capitalist societies, where discourses of choice, freedom, and autonomy coexist ... alongside the proliferation of highly restrictive and regulatory discourses of hypersexualized femininity" (p. 314). This depiction is rooted in a version of North American sexual history wherein the "first" sexual revolution of the 1960s and 1970s, spawned by medical technologies such as "the pill," are seen to have uncoupled heterosex from reproduction and morality, rendering it an equal playing field for all genders and identities.

Such representations of women's heterosexual freedom ignore the ways in which the sexual double standard persists, a point well documented in empirical research. As just a small sample of this literature, surveys of US college students from 1965 to 1985 demonstrate the ongoing stigmatization of women's promiscuity and the normalization of men's (for a summary of some of these surveys, see Robinson, Ziss, Ganza, Katz, & Robinson, 1991). Hite's (1976) nationwide survey of women in the United Kingdom about their sexuality led her to conclude: "Women who did try to be open and share with men, having sex in the new, free way, in all too many cases would end up being disrespected and often hurt – because the double standard is still operating" (p. 468). The Women, Risk, and AIDS Protection (WRAP) team of researchers' interviews with hundreds of British youth from 1988 to 1990 reveal the ongoing strength of the sexual double standard. The team notes "behaviour that made him successfully masculine, a real man, caused her to lose her reputation – to be seen as loose, slack, a slag – a reputation policed just as forcefully by women as by men" (Holland et al., 1998, p. 11).

However, the WRAP team also notes a common factor among the young women in their study that might set them apart from women their age in previous decades, and might be a persistent feature of het-erosex for many women today. The researchers argue that both the young women and young men they interviewed were governed by "the male in the head." In this paradigm, "heterosexuality is not, as it appears to be, masculinity-and-femininity in opposition, *it is mascu-linity*" (Holland et al., 1999, p. 11, emphasis added). According to the WRAP researchers, the masculine model, which governs heterosexual norms, informs the expectations, meanings, and practices of those in the heterosexual contract. Understanding masculinity as a hegemonic ideal, which governs through an internalized "male gaze," helps us make sense of women's active participation in aspects of heterosexual culture that do not seem to benefit many women socially or sexually.

Although autobiographical anthologies such as *Jane Sexes It Up: True Confessions of Feminist Desire* (Johnson, 2002) are a testament to the full and pleasurable sex lives of many women in the so-called third wave of feminism, a substantial body of research concludes that young women in particular continue to struggle to prioritize and realize their own heterosexual desires and pleasures on an experiential level, even when claiming to feel empowered. Tolman (2001) argues that "female sexual adolescent dysfunction is an oxymoron," since her empirical research suggests that "teenage girls would meet the [*Diagnostic and Statisti-cal Manual of Mental Disorders*] criteria for sexual dysfunction" more often than not. Despite the intense sexualization of young women, her research has led to her conclude that "it is still not 'normal,' not acceptable ... for girls to believe that they can or should have their own sexual desire and pleasure" (p. 197). Although all of the above refers to consensual heterosexual intercourse, Gavey's (1993, 2005) research reminds us of the normalization of rape culture in popular discourse.

Recent examinations of the gender politics of adult sexuality simi-larly complicate post-feminist notions of "reciprocal" heterosex sex as a gender-neutral, equal exchange of sexual effort for orgasm (Gilfoyle, Wilson, & Own, 1992). As Braun, Gavey, and McPhillips (2003) argue, women are expected to deliver orgasms, both their own and their part-ner's. And yet, whereas men's orgasms are for the most part seen as integral to heterosex, women's are often seen as a "bonus" (Roberts, Kippax, Waldby, & Crawford, 1995). Moreover, as Gavey (1993) states, "To say that [adult] women often engage in unwanted sex with men is paradoxically both to state the obvious and to speak the unmentionable" (p. 93). Although none of the above research takes an explicitly intersectional lens – as, for example, Skeggs (1997) does in her book, *Formations of Class and Gender: Becoming Respectable* – race, class, ability, and other intersecting aspects of identity also shape the construction, experience, and judgment of one's sexuality (Crenshaw, 1989).

### Reflections on Early Heterosex

> People learn when they are quite young a few things that are expected to be, and continue slowly to accumulate a belief in who they are and ought to be through the rest of childhood, adolescence, and adulthood. Sexual conduct is learned in the same way and through the same processes: it is acquired and assembled through human interaction, judged and performed in specific cultural and historical worlds. (Gagnon, 1977, p. 2)

Although demonstrating a clear ability to engage critically with the discursive fields they came into contact with, the participants in my study pinpointed several media as influencing their perceptions and experiences of sexuality. Sarah, a student in her twenties, commented on the influence of popular culture in endorsing a very narrow vision of being sexual, as embodied in white, blonde, thin women such as Britney Spears. She lamented, "What does to be sexy mean? To be sexy is purely visual these days." Simone, a thirty-year-old sex worker, commented, "It's everywhere in all our forms of entertainment and everything we're sold. And so many people don't fit into that." Louise, a single parent, claimed that "every single individual" is affected by the dominance of certain definitions of sexuality, but "girls are more attuned to it."

Women in this study cited mainstream heterosexual pornography as having a major influence on them at a young age, albeit in very different ways.[1] Reflecting on her introduction to porn as a young woman in South Africa, thirty-four-year-old Anna stated, "It was just imprinted on me that I am there to give pleasure or pleasure myself, but that I'm not going to be the recipient ... That's sort of come into my sexual imagining or whatever you call it when you become sexualized." Maria, twenty-two, felt that the mainstream heterosexual porn that she and her partners used as sex education had a reverberating effect. Of her male partners' relationship with porn, she stated, "As soon as they got the Internet, they were fiends. And all they saw were skinny girls with boob jobs doing things that a lot of girls wouldn't want to do in the real world. It kind of ruined them." She also wondered if the fact that women in porn seemingly "get off so fast" sends an unrealistic message.

It might seem old-fashioned to talk about "peer pressure," but this term came up often in discussions of early heterosex. The women in my study cited the influence of peers and partners in their teenage years as key agents of sexual socialization. Lauren, the youngest woman in the study at age twenty-one, recited a poem she wrote: "There seems to be a stigma against virgins … Everyone tells me I need to take care of my little problem. My problem. What my problem is, is trying to find someone to trust. Not a prude. Not innocent. Not afraid." In another instance, she specifically pinpointed pressure from girlfriends, claiming, "For all their coercion, you know, like 'You've just got to let it go! It's not that big a deal!' Deep down something made me know I didn't want that." These sentiments highlight Carpenter's (2002) theory that, for young women now, as it has long been for young men, losing one's virginity is a matter of shedding the stigma of not being sexually active.

There was also general consensus among these heterosexual women that male partners held more authority in setting heterosexual norms from the beginning. Once the majority of the women in the study were initiated into sexual relationships involving intercourse, they identified these early relationships as favouring men's sexual needs over their own. Several of the women used the term "selfish" to describe the sexual approach taken by teenage boys. Of her first long-term sexual relationship, Maria claimed "It felt like as soon as he got one taste of the genital [pause], he was just a fiend for it." She later added, "That's all he cared about. He didn't care about kissing me or anything. He didn't care about touching my breasts. He only cared about that one area." She concluded, "For guys, it's about getting, not giving. On every level, it's not fair. They have the pleasure and we don't."

A striking one-fifth of participants from a range of self-described social locations had experienced sexual abuse as a child, and discussed this history as having had a direct influence on their future experience of heterosex. Zoe, a thirty-four-year-old white Canadian radio documentary maker, described being "simultaneously sexually abused by my mother's husband and my stepbrother" as "vaguely" influencing her sexual experiences. Jolene, a fifty-one-year-old indigenous woman, recalled her first sexual experience as "being a little kid … my uncle George was trying to molest me." Celia, a fifty-six-year-old Chinese-Canadian nurse, recalled sexual abuse by an uncle as leaving a "traumatic impression" on her views of sex. Maria (Italian-Canadian) and Jas (Indo-Canadian) both identified the legacy of child sexual abuse in terms similar to those Anna used in describing the impression that watching porn as a child made on her. They explained child sexual abuse as "conditioning" their awareness of men's sexual needs and their perceived duty to satisfy "the male sex drive" (Hollway, 1984). For instance, Jas, who was raped by her uncle from ages five to fifteen, described her present relationships with men by stating, "I can automatically understand how the other person feels. I'm very much into what they're feeling. It's the result of much conditioning." When discussing her reaction to being sexually abused as a child by her grandfather, Maria claimed, "Whether I really want to or not, I always respond to sexual tension … So, it's kind of like being obligated."

The women discussed numerous instances of sexual violence and coercion when recounting adolescence. Lauren, a young, white, middle-class woman, considered herself "very lucky" for managing to avoid "getting myself raped": "I've had experiences where I almost *got myself raped* last year because of a situation where saying 'no' angered someone. You know he didn't actually do anything to me and *luckily* I was able to leave … he started pushing my comfort zone. I was going, 'Keep your underwear on. I don't want them to come off.' And he's like, 'Fine! If you don't want me to pleasure you and you don't want to pleasure me,' and he started getting really angry" (emphasis added). While violence against women spans all social classes, Lauren's social capital in relation to race and class may have played a role in her supposed "luck" in this instance.

In addition to everyday structural and other forms of violence, indigenous women in Canada face at least triple the rate of sexual violence that non-indigenous women do (Brennan, 2011). Jolene, the indigenous woman, depicted her early sexual experiences as being a continuum of male violence. She recalled her sexual experiences as a youth:

> I've been physically assaulted, verbally assaulted, sexually assaulted on a number of occasions. I couldn't begin to count the date rapes. I was in one situation, when I was a very young teenager, a girl and I were hitchhiking, two guys picked us up. We basically got kidnapped. She put out for both

of us and they basically left me alone. I remember being held down by a boyfriend who I really cared for. He and his buddy came over and they held me down and they both raped me. Date rapes – many. Having sex when I didn't want to – most of the time.

Although indigenous women have actively resisted all forms of violence, the construction of the "squaw" as a colonial strategy for sexualizing, conflating, and dehumanizing their identities operates to normalize and excuse these instances of violence (Razack, 2000). When taking into consideration violence associated with colonization, patriarchy, and capitalism, biomedical notions of sexual dysfunction as an individual, internal problem seem particularly reductionist.

### Talking about Adult Heterosex

When reflecting on adult heterosex, participants depicted ongoing coercive pressure to conform to normative heterosexual ideals. Although the majority described learning about compulsory intercourse as teenagers, five middle-aged women from religious backgrounds claimed not to feel pressure to engage in coital penetration until marriage. After describing the sense of pride she felt about her early decisions regarding premarital abstinence, Olivia, a thirty-seven-year-old Mexican-Canadian woman explained, "But then we were married and it was like, 'Well if you're married, you have sex.' … Whereas before it was considered to be acceptable to engage in what is considered as foreplay, marriage required getting out of that pattern." Celia, a Chinese-Canadian woman, recalled the details of her sex life when she was married, stating, "I just engaged in sexual activity with him out of the goodness of my heart so to speak. And then I know, after having sex, then I know he wouldn't bother with me for three days." She later added, "I didn't realize what my sexual pattern was until he would go away on a business trip. Maybe not even going for four days or even a week at the most. Then I would dread him coming home because I would have to have sex. Sort of obligatory sex."

Studies suggest that women who are unable to engage in intercourse due to chronic genital pain, or do not orgasm as a result of intercourse more generally, often feel like "unreal" women (Kaler, 2006; Lavie & Willig, 2005; Lavie-Ayjayi & Joffe, 2009; Nicolson & Burr, 2003), a finding that was paralleled in my interviews. Participants who could not or would not take part in regular penetrative sex often faced direct consequences, such as male frustration, anger, and/or coercion and abuse. Maria described an ex-boyfriend's reaction to her lack of sexual desire in her adult years, stating, "He was just really scarring and emotionally scarring, emotionally abusive. And I already recognized that he'd be mad at me if I didn't feel like having sex. He'd make me feel bad about it." Zoe revealed that, when her interest in sexual intercourse waned, her partner began a campaign to make her jealous. She explained: "So I got to hear about all the girls who were attractive and what type of women he was into. And the fact that my legs weren't long enough and my breasts weren't big enough. And why didn't I wear this and why didn't I wear that?" Louise described her partner's mood changes when she withheld sex for a certain amount of time, confiding, "He gets frustrated and kind of acts out about it and then he's over it." But "if we don't have sex in a week ... or a two-week period, it's just hell. He'll be sarcastic and make comments, like little jokes. He'll say, 'What's the difference?'" These comments demonstrate the consequences faced by women who do not take part in the most expected sexual activity, sexual intercourse, and also reveal their resentment towards their partners' punitive measures.

Those who refused or were unable to have penetrative sex were also aware that they risked being left by male partners, a point they described matter-of-factly. As a woman with little sexual interest or desire, Kate, a forty-four-year-old stay-at-home mother, was frank about the role of compulsory sex in sustaining her marriage. She admitted that not having unwanted intercourse every now and then would mean that "I would probably be divorced." Elizabeth, a fifty-seven-year-old retired counsellor, claimed that "giving up on sex ... would be bad for the marriage." Charlene bluntly admitted, "He's told me that's why maybe we're not married." Her partner regularly asks her: "How many times a day can you jerk off?" Linda, a pre-medical-school student, became aware of the threat of being dumped through the experiences of other women. She recalled her initiation into online sexual support groups for women with sexual pain, stating, "I remember, when I first joined, all they could talk about was divorcing their husbands, or husbands treating them like crap, or husbands feeling they need to cheat on their wives"; she concluded, "that was really depressing to hear about." Mika, a twenty-seven-year-old bookstore employee, explained how her partner of four years broke up with her due to his "biological urge to thrust." She mused: "We were still being intimate in other ways. Doing "everything but," but then "he would pull away. He didn't want to fool around anymore because he found it too frustrating, so we weren't having any kind of sexual contact at all." She described the breakup as "a huge, huge, thing" and felt "a lot of sadness about him because" she "really felt like he was 'the one'" and they "were so good together as a couple."

For single women with sexual problems, the fear was not of being dumped, but of never finding a long-term companion in the first place. Lindsay, a thirty-nine-year-old nurse who had "problems" with sexual desire and arousal, straightforwardly equated her distress over sexual difficulties with the difficulty of finding a life partner. Her tone was frank when discussing the centrality of intercourse in heterosexual relationships and her awareness of this cultural norm. She explained, "it never goes past one to three months ... simply because my lack of libido obviously plays a role. Men want to feel like they can stimulate a partner. I'm not stimulated. Obviously, that makes them feel inadequate, and so the relationship dissolves." In a similar vein, Courtney, a student diagnosed with vaginismus, bitterly recalled, "It got to the point where I was concerned that I wouldn't find someone." As she stated, "For a long time, I just dated virgins, thinking naively, 'They're not going to want to have sex!' But university guys are a little bit different." Mika reflected on being a newly single woman with chronic genital pain, stating, "my biggest fear right now is I do obviously want a companion one day and I want to be able to have sex with somebody. But besides that, in the absence of that, I hope there is somebody who will want to be with me anyways."

Given all of these pressures to conform to heteronormative ideals, it is no surprise that, for some women, their sexual problems led to a questioning of their identity as "real" or "healthy" women.' Danielle, a forty-four-year-old married teacher who identifies as having chronic genital pain, claimed that, for years, her inability to have coital sex had made her feel like "an android," not "a real woman." Danielle said she felt she could not "perform what I see as the sexual acts that women do." Similarly, through tears, Sophie, a thirty-two-year-old British student, described feeling "foolish" and as though she was "disappointing men" because she was not able to "do a pretty basic thing that a woman should be able to do." She later added, "I get concerned about letting people down. Like disappointing men if I'm not able to fulfil certain expectations or do all the activities. Olivia, who told me that she thought labelling someone as "frigid" was "horrible," contradictorily also claimed that her "whole life has been a waste of time" because of her inability to have penetrative sex.

## Sharing Heterosexual Inadequacy: Secrecy and Confession

Judging by neoliberal, post-feminist media such as the television show *Sex and the City*, one might imagine that heterosexual women collectively confide in other women about their sexual anxieties and problems on a regular basis. But the majority of the participants in this study claimed not to confide in their friends about their sex lives, and described an intense need to uphold a normative image to their peers. This was true of participants of all ages, social classes, and ethnic backgrounds. Women from a range of ethnic backgrounds cited their "culture" as getting in the way. Monica, a Chinese-Canadian yoga teacher in her forties, perceived her hesitance to confide in friends as a cultural issue. She stated, "I think my culture gets in there. [In Chinese culture] you don't ask people how much money they make and you don't talk about sex." However, several women made the same comments about their white European backgrounds, which they referred to as "repressed" or "WASPy."

Julie, a twenty-seven-year-old office manager, explained that her friends regularly talked about "sexual politics," "relationship problems that aren't related to sex," or "how sexually attractive" they think someone is, but not "the mechanics of sexual problems." Celia never confided in her friends about her lack of sexual enjoyment, stating, "I didn't feel I could because ... when my husband and I were at parties, they would say, 'Oh! What a lovely couple you are!'" She feared jeopardizing this image of successful heterosexuality. Faye speculated that this was a common sentiment among women because "there's so much competition between women. You just don't go there because you've got to seem like you've got it all together." Nicola, a thirty-four-year-old teacher, also rued, "It could have been the stress of not wanting your friends to think your relationship is sucking. It could be the female competition, you know?" Similarly, Zoe lamented, "none of our friends ... know that we have such terrible difficulties. It's embarrassing. I feel that I'm not servicing my partner." Olivia was distrustful of her friends, claiming she had never once mentioned to a single friend that her sixteen-year marriage was "unconsummated." Other than her doctors, I was the first person she had told. Through tears, she commented,

"It's just [that], you know, people judge. I mean maybe I can deal with me, but I don't want anybody to be saying bad things about my husband … or them telling me, 'What, are you stupid?' Because I know that is what they would say … It's too humiliating."

Although the women in this study were cautious about admitting to their friends that their sex lives did not measure up to the societal gold standard, they relished the rare opportunities to talk to female strangers who shared their experiences. Particularly for women with sexual pain, support groups were another way to temper the alienation they felt from their friends and partners. Six participants attended grassroots support groups regularly – three of them were part of the support group for chronic sexual pain described in the previous chapter. This group met once a month to share stories and exchange information and advice. Four of the six women who were in grassroots support groups also participated in two different Yahoo online "support groups" for women with sexual pain issues. Susan, sixty-two, was a member of a menopausal support group that touched on sexual issues. Regular lay support groups attended by women facing similar issues gave participants the sense of collectivity they craved.

Participants also described unexpected support through grassroots workshops that did not specifically cater to women experiencing sexual problems. Both Lauren and Courtney were involved in a university production of *The Vagina Monologues*, and took part in mandatory workshops for all cast and crew at which attendees were asked to explore cultural silence and stigma around vulvas and vaginas. Lauren viewed these workshops as a form of "self-counselling" and central to her "getting over" her fear and anxiety surrounding her body and sexual interactions. Courtney, a twenty-five year old university administrator, had a similar experience as a director and former actor in this production.[2]

Simone took part in a grassroots workshop specifically organized for sex workers. Over the course of a month-long workshop, participants lived together in Vancouver and then on a nearby island. This retreat was sponsored by the Access to Media Education Society, an organization that uses film making as therapy for various groups. Participants took part in daily sessions sharing their experiences of paid sex work and related issues and made a documentary about the sex trade. She described the film project as "helping us to explore our feelings, patterns, that kind of thing." She explained, "We just looked at ourselves and our bodies," adding "It was really interesting but was really intensive just dealing with each other's stuff." In her reference to "each other's stuff," the isolation of sexual difficulties seems to have broken down once sexual problems were reconceptualized as a collective issue. She claimed, "We were really supportive of each other. And I came out of that feeling really inspired and kind of empowered and … whether I do this or not I'm just going to feel good about it."

### Heteronormativity in Non-heterosexual Relationships?

Are non-heterosexual relationships and interactions necessarily without the normative trappings of heteronormativity, or are the pressures of heteronormativity more difficult to escape than that? Clearly, with only one self-identified lesbian participant, three bisexual participants (one of whom listed herself as bisexual but never commented on her attraction to women), and absolutely no participants who identified as queer, gender queer, and/or trans*, my small sample was limited. If anything, as discussed in the following chapter, my study has deconstructed the work of adhering to gender and sexual normativity. And even if I were to have a more representative sample, as Plummer (2007) argues, those who attempt to construct "universal homosexuals," or any universal identity, "striding round history and across cultures simply miss the importance of precarious and contingent social organization" (p. 24). With these significant points acknowledged, comments of the few participants who discussed same-sex relationships offer some possible insight for future debates on the issue of heteronormativity as a hegemonic ideal.

To a certain degree, same-sex sexual relationships were described as offering refuge from normative heterosexuality. Leanne, the only self-identified lesbian in the study, did not like "the implied heterosexuality" of the book *For Women Only: A Revolutionary Guide to Reclaiming Your Sex Life* (Berman et al., 2001). She viewed herself as being more sexually aware than her straight counterparts, and believed, "There are probably a lot of straight housewives who are running around the suburbs who need help, but I'm not in that category." She also identified female sexual relationships as involving less pressure, stating, "There wasn't that same issue about intercourse." She argued that men tend to be sexually more goal-oriented than women, and concluded, "It's kind of a relief to be with a woman partner" and "Women don't have as much at stake."

Although Leanne might have viewed women sexual partners as having a more fluid approach to sexuality, notions of sexual "normality" seemed to be still part of her way of thinking. She herself was arguably one of the most distressed and goal-oriented participants in the study. Her quest to orgasm was apparently fuelled largely by her "embarrassment" over "being dysfunctional." These feelings had led her to use vibrators so vigorously that, in her opinion, she had damaged the nerve endings of her clitoris. As evidence of her goal-oriented outlook, she commented, "So, … what I call dysfunctional is that I can't *guarantee* [orgasm]. So, it's a really emotional thing for me. It's really traumatic." She later reflected, "For a while I just had casual affairs where I didn't feel that pressured because I wouldn't see these people again and I didn't care. That way I could still have sex but it didn't have to be about that … I'm still not in a place where I'm really comfortable. I'm not confident that I'll orgasm every time, and that's hard to live with. You know to my partner, I have to often say, 'Are you sure we want to do this tonight?'" Contrary to her own self-perception of having a distinct and developed sexual outlook, Leanne's comments on the "trauma" of being "dysfunctional," defined as being unable to "guarantee" orgasm, reflect a normative understanding of sex. Although she might have challenged the notion of "compulsory heterosexuality," she had not questioned the notion of compulsory orgasm.

The very small sample of bisexual participants commented that they were disappointed to find that certain gender roles and attitudes towards sex replicated themselves in same-sex sexual relationships. As a self-proclaimed femme, Zoe pointed to the implications of butch/femme roles in some same-sex partnerships. When discussing her orgasm problems, she stated, "I think, when you're having sex with women, I mean, it is really bizarre to me that the whole gender roles get played out in gay relationships where there's the butch and the femme. And it was just amazing to me that that existed once I got in there." Simone felt having sexual relationships with women re-enacted traditional masculine and feminine gender roles and involved pressures similar to those in heterosexual relationships. When discussing her recent lack of sexual desire, she claimed, "I can still feel really screwed up with a woman and I can still bring in all those weird identity kinds of questions and that sort of confusion … I feel as a result of the media and some stereotypes … I find that, just because I'm with a woman, it doesn't make it go away." Simone's comments suggest that, whether she is in a relationship with a woman or a man, she confronts dominant norms or "stereotypes" of sex and gender.[3]

These sentiments defy radical feminist literature – for example, Jeffreys (1990, 1994); Rich (1980) – which assumes that same-sex sexuality necessarily challenges the heteronormative paradigm. They support more recent arguments that heteronormativity has not "relinquished its hegemonic hold" on the experiences of gays and lesbians (Richardson, 1996, p. 3) and that lesbian and bisexual women also must negotiate expectations associated with normative heterosexuality (Jackson, 1999). They are in keeping with Stein's (2009) perhaps obvious remark that "the boundaries separating the group called 'lesbians' from the rest of women are not at all clearly or immutably marked" (p. 93).

## Conclusions

Although advocates of sexual pharmaceuticals have attempted to locate sexual dissatisfaction in the vascular, hormonal, and neuroscientific arena, several social factors seem to limit women's potential for experiencing sexual pleasure. Chief among these are the narrow confines of socially defined "normal" or "successful" heterosex. According to the participants in my study, female friends, male partners, popular culture, and pornography are influential agents of socialization into sexual norms. These agents by and large construct and celebrate a narrow heterosexual script within a very particular vision of sexiness. The accounts of participants demonstrate the role of macro power systems such as patriarchy, colonialism, and capitalism in shaping their sexual difficulties.

Participants' recollections of early sexual experiences were marked by the immediacy of pressure to engage in coitus as the hallowed act of heterosex, a perceived lack of control over the choice of whether or not to have sexual relations, and a sense of disappointment accompanying early heterosex. A significant number of these women described internalizing the pressure to meet certain sexual expectations as a result of childhood experiences – for example, early exposure to mainstream heterosexual pornography or child sexual abuse. Their reflections on early and adult experiences of heterosexuality suggest that male partners were often coercive, pursuing sexual acts when women were not enjoying them, at times not taking "no" for an answer, expressing anger and frustration, and threatening to leave if the woman did not meet normative heterosexual standards. Many identified sexual power relations with notable tones of resentment and disappointment.

Indicative of the tensions and contradictions of what some see as the "post-feminist" era (Braithwaite, 2002) – despite many participants' low self esteem and disappointment that they did not match up to the heterosexual gold standard – the women in my study revealed a high degree of consciousness and reflexivity about the constraining nature of heteronormativity. When reflecting on their early and/or adult heterosexual experiences, they matter-of-factly detailed gender-based relationship inequalities, violence, and coercion, often expressing disappointment with the limited repertoire that normative heterosex demands. Their accounts described the prevalence of normative expectations and, in some cases, the violence used to compel women to accept men as partners. They also indicated an astute awareness of heterosexuality, and sexuality more generally, as compulsory.

Unfortunately, awareness of the pressure of heterosexuality did not seem to lessen its bite. Despite feeling comfortable about discussing narratives of sexual pleasure with friends, the women in my study were less likely to discuss non-pleasurable sexual experiences with women in their personal lives. But, in the face of this shared awareness of the constraints associated with normative sexuality, some were working actively to meeting heterosexual standards, as I examine in the next chapter, while others were challenging these standards, as I discuss in Chapter 5.

# 4 Sex Work: A Labour of Love

I expected that the women in this study would access a wide range of services and tools with a view to sexual improvement. I imagined some of these services and tools would be exclusive, expensive, and medicalized, while others would be accessible, inexpensive, and originate from grassroots demedicalized or non-medicalized sources. To a certain extent, this prediction proved correct: for women with the privilege of access to sexual advice in an urban, cosmopolitan city such as Vancouver, the options are numerous. The majority of the women in this study accessed some kind of professional advice or therapy, whether in a face-to-face professional setting or in the context of self-help. In theory, advice from general practitioners (GPs), gynecologists, and sexual medicine specialists, as well as access to group therapy and support groups, was available through British Columbia's health care insurance free of direct cost. But, although public sector resources are supposedly "free," they take perseverance and social capital to pursue. And private sector services such as pelvic physiotherapy, sex therapy, counselling, naturopathy, massage therapy, acupuncture, and commercial goods such as sex toys and sex manuals come at a direct price. Thus, access to professional and commercial services for sexual improvement is a largely, though not strictly, a middle-class option in the Canadian context.

When considering these diverse sources, however, I once again came to discern a common thread: the overall goal of most types of therapies, whether medicalized, demedicalized, or never medicalized in the first place, was by and large to working towards changing a woman's sexual response to meet sexual norms in some way – "the labour of love," as I have come to see it. In this chapter, I consider evidence of the "work" the women in my study were willing to undertake to resolve the contradictions they experienced in heteronormative expectations and realities. I develop the concept of unpaid "sex work," a term coined by Duncombe and Marsden (1996) to conceptualize women's engagement with the rationalization, improvement, and mastery of sexual pleasure in personal sexual relationships. In the only other qualitative interview study examining sex work in intimate heterosexual relationships, these authors found that "most emotion (and by analogy sex) work will be undertaken by women" (p. 222). Sex work has parallels with "emotional work" (Hochschild, 1983), including many forms of invisible care-giving by women (Twigg et al., 2011), naturalized as part of the heterosexual division of labour.

I am not the first to point out that sexuality is a prime candidate for hard work and managerial attention. Jackson and Scott (1997) have highlighted the rationalization and even "Taylorization" of sex (p. 558) in a "post-Fordist" society (p. 564), leading to a trend that Harvey and Gill (2011) have referred to as "intimate entrepreneurship" (p. 3). But while these sources consider the role of self-help and popular advice to women in promoting sex work, my work considers these sources on a continuum with the sex work advocated by highly medicalized sources and demedicalized grassroots approaches.

I also demonstrate distinctions between kinds of sex work using a schema of discipline work, performance work, and avoidance work. Sexual advice practitioners, both those whom I interviewed or observed and those described by interview participants, advocated women's discipline work as essential for the survival of relationships. This is not surprising given the normalization of women's emotional and sexual labour, but also given that the careers of these professionals depend on the ongoing popularity of disciplining the body for sexual enjoyment.

### Historicizing the Sex Work Imperative

It is almost difficult to imagine that expert sex advice in Anglo-Western texts was once primarily aimed at men. As Bullough (1973) notes, sex manuals dating back to medieval times had an assumed heterosexual male audience. They offered detailed information about women's bodies in the spirit that men's understanding women's anatomy would be useful for procreation and mutual pleasure. Marriage manuals of the early twentieth century continued to call on men to hone their sexual skills. Neuhaus (2000) references works by Havelock Ellis (1913), Paul

Popenoe (1925), Theodore H. Van de Velde (1930), and C.B.S. Evans (1931) as examples of texts extolling men to work on their sexual technique.

*Harmony in Marriage* by Leland Foster Wood and Robert Latou Dickinson (1939) is another case in point. The section on "Physical Harmony" focuses on advice to husbands on how to make sex more comfortable and enjoyable for their wives. In a section on "Faults of Sexual Approach," they write: "By wrong approach, the husband may fail to make the marital relationship a means of charming and delighting his wife, but rather may repel her. With a demanding rather than love making attitude, he neglects to bring his wife's sexual emotions into life. From ignorance he passes through a sequence of haste and clumsiness, causing pain, and even aversion. This can be remedied by attention to the woman's needs and the ways of satisfying them as we have discussed" (p. 68). When discussing sexual difficulties, the main focus is how men can delay ejaculation to provide more time for women to reach orgasm. Wood and Dickinson write:

> He may experience a quick ejaculation of the seminal fluid, after which he may be unable to bring his wife to her orgasm. Since the wife's emotional tide naturally rises more slowly, it is only by delaying his orgasm that the husband will be able to completely satisfy her. To learn this may take time, but he will think of his love, rather than fears, and in the course of the experience will discover the positions and movements which bring his wife to her culmination while enabling him to delay his own. (pp. 68–9)

It is fair to say that their writings are steeped in essentialist and binary views of gender and sexuality. Unlike contemporary expert advice on sex, however, Wood and Dickinson place the onus of successful heterosex on men.

By the 1950s, the intended audience for expert sexual advice found in marriage manuals had changed dramatically. Mid-century manuals such as *Modern Woman: The Lost Sex* (Lundberg, 1947), *The Psychology of Women* (Deutsch, 1944), *How To Hold Your Husband: Frank Psychoanalysis for Happy Marriage* (Gill, 1951), and *Responsibility in Marriage* (Davis, 1963) were aimed at women. They ignored the possibility of faulty male sexual technique, rather blaming women for their own failure to experience pleasure. These texts reveal the influence of Freudian ideas about psychosexual development, particularly the view that vaginal orgasm represents female sexual maturity, and clitoral orgasm sexual immaturity. But the sexual labour expected of women in these texts was not purely physical. Books such as *A Marriage Doctor Speaks Her Mind about Sex* warned, "It is important for a man to have a loving and understanding wife. If she gives him confidence in himself, he will be able to perform adequately" (Liswood & Davis, 1961, quoted in Neuhaus, 2000, p. 60). Here we see an example of how sex work is part and parcel of women's emotional as well as physical management of relationships.

Free-love theorist Herbert Marcuse (1955) once argued that prioritizing sexual pleasure could be an explicitly anticapitalist, antiproductive, and rebellious act. But many have noted that the tenets associated with the "sexual revolution" were hijacked by commercial, capitalist interests, as "sex sells" advertising and a sexual marketplace began to flourish (Erenreich & English, 1978; Hawkes, 1996). As part of the booming commodification of sex, expert sexual advice exploded, particularly via pop psychology and sexual self-help aimed at women via therapy groups, television talk shows, sex manuals, and magazine articles.

Upon first glance, post-sexual revolution discourses on sexual improvement appeared liberating to women. Backed by scientific sexological research by Masters and Johnson (1966) and Kaplan (1977), there was increasing acceptance of the notion that women are as sexual as men and that clitoral orgasm is far more common than vaginal. In a barrage of self-help advice, women were told that if they "unlearn their socialization and imitate male style" (Masters & Johnson, p. 308), anyone could express themselves sexually without consequence. Feminist critics have highlighted the paradox of this period for women as, in theory, some women were given licence to exercise sexual freedom, but to a large extent this was dependent on age, race, and class (Skeggs, 1997). Further, women faced more intense pressure than ever to be sexy, sexual, and good at sex (Erenreich & English, 1978; Jeffreys, 1990). Helen Gurley Brown, author of *Sex and the Single Girl* (1962) and editor of *Cosmopolitan* magazine, called upon young women to "transform their apartments into lairs of erotic fascination" (Ehrenreich & English, 1978, p. 287), and fashion their bodies for feminine seduction. As Jeffries (1997) argues, whereas the spinster of decades previous would have taken comfort in her intelligence or her relationships with friends, the new single girl was chiefly responsible for the "stimulation of the male sexual appetite" (p. 107).

Within this context of compulsory sexuality, sexual capital has taken on new value alongside and intertwined with economic, cultural, and social capital (Bordieu, 1984), particularly for women. Sexual capital is often overlooked in discussions of power and privilege, but it is particularly important for those with less economic, cultural, and social capital, women included. According to Hakim (2010), "erotic capital" is defined by elements such as beauty, attractiveness, social grace and charm, liveliness, style, fertility, and "sexuality itself: sexual competence, energy, erotic imagination, playfulness and everything else that makes for a sexually satisfying partner" (p. 499). Hakim's work is explicitly antifeminist, drawing on evolutionary biology to explain the overemphasis on women's sexual traits as necessary for human reproduction. I use the term "sexual capital" to distance myself from Hakim's essentialist theorizing of gender, the erotic, and reproduction. I also note that Hakim's definition of erotic capital is based entirely on factors related to pleasing one's partner(s). The findings I report in Chapter 3 suggest, however, that a woman's own capacity for sexual pleasure is as integral a part of her sexual capital as her ability to please her partner sexually. Heterosexual women who lack desire or have difficulty with arousal, orgasm, or penetration face a serious drop in their sexual capital.

Although I agree with the potential of recognizing sexual enjoyment as a "talent" that can be a personal strength, or honed with a little attention, as Tiefer (2004) has argued, it is important to examine who is targeted to do the work of heterosexual improvement and who feels compelled to do it. Women are still two-thirds of the purchasers of self-help guides in the category of "relationship" and "family" (Blakeley, 2009) and more likely to seek professional advice for anything "health" related, as sex is now considered to be. This kind of advice exhorts women to take care of both their own sexual problems and their partner's, "being [sic] supportive-massaging egos and sometimes the penis itself" (Jackson & Scott, 1997, p. 53). As Tyler (2004) notes, the work mandate is particularly prevalent in women's magazines, exhorting women to hone their "performance imperative" (p. 97), promoting a "rationalized," "colonized," and even "McDonaldized" sexual experience (p. 99). As examples, she offers quotes such as "train yourself for really ambitious sex"; "guaranteed – the best sex ever"; "great sex – 20 ways to perfect your style"; and "how to achieve world class love making." As Gupta and I have argued (2013), even when sex work is aimed at a seemingly gender-neutral audience in popular sex manuals, it is often subtly gendered as an instruction for women. As I show in the next chapter, material factors also constrain women's sense of options and choices for refusing to do the work of sexual improvement.

## The Work of Sexual Improvement

I have identified three distinct types of sex work – discipline work, performance work, and avoidance work – involving physical and psychological work on participants' own bodies and minds and those of their sexual partners. Participants who identified as having various sexual difficulties had tried different types of sex work at certain stages of their lives for a range of reasons. Discipline work refers to sex work aimed at changing one's mental and physical sexual response to standard heterosexual sexual practices. By contrast, performance work entails "faking it" using a range of techniques, while avoidance work involves evading the issue all together employing a number of strategies.

Discipline work is characterized by the quest to implement a certain skill and/or degree of concentration to manipulate the body or the mind. Therefore, participants who had consulted GPs, gynecologists, psychologists, psychiatrists, sexual medicine specialists, pelvic physiotherapists, marriage counsellors, sex therapists, naturopaths, and New Age healers had been advised to discipline the way they respond to sexual prompts. Thus, participants who had tried pills, creams, gels, herbal remedies, vaginal dilators, dildos, and vibrators to improve their sex lives had taken part in discipline work. Those who had sought information from books, magazines, the Internet, friends, and partners about how to change their mental and physical sexual response similarly had been implicated in this type of work. In the service of discipline work, therefore, participants had allowed their bodies to be examined, monitored, assessed, and touched in the most intimate ways. Participants' overall attitude, whether or not they saw themselves as sexually dysfunctional, was that they could hone skills such as discipline, concentration, and focus that would alter their response to heteronormative sex. This type of work seemed to demand long-term commitment because it is time consuming. Participants with perceived sexual problems and the practitioners I interviewed were of the firm belief that the less the commitment by the couple, the less likely would the partner be willing to remain in the relationship, join in the work, or wait patiently while the woman independently tried to improve the sexual aspects of their relationship. These findings are in contrast to Duncombe and Marsden's (1996) suggestion that, "unfortunately, it seems to be only relatively briefly (before marriage)" that partners are prepared to do sex work.

As Duncombe and Marsden (1996) remind us, "sex work may be either fulfilling or distasteful, depending upon the relational context in which it is performed" (p. 235). Some participants described discipline work in terms of "getting to know myself sexually" or "learning about my sexuality." In other words, it is possible that they had constructed and reaffirmed their sexual identities through sex work as well as enjoying the process of exploring their sexuality. As we saw in Chapter 2, women with chronic sexual pain were positive about many aspects of disciplining sex (in these cases hetero) sex. Aside from their grievances about the cost and accessibility of professionally led body-work therapies, they viewed them in empowering terms. Since most of these women had been told at some point that their sexual pain was "all in their heads," and had been generally "ignored" or "dismissed" by the medical profession or approached with a heavy hand, they appreciated being taken seriously and the gentle but "hands-on" attention they received during sexual medicine and pelvic physiotherapy treatments. They felt the process of disciplining mind and body through visual aids such as mirrors or biofeedback increased their sense of control and awareness of their own bodies. As Mika stated, "to have the actual feedback was very helpful ... You could feel your body relaxing and you see it happening and so as a result you're in better control of it."

Turning to performance work, Duncombe and Marsden (1996) found that women in long-term relationships took part in what the authors refer to as "playing the couple game," denoting a cycle common to long-term "fading" heterosexual relationships wherein women "deep act" away feelings of doubt, presenting the image of "the happy couple" before "leaking" criticisms about their relationship to outsiders (p. 221). Duncombe and Marsden (1996) and Jackson and Scott (2001) have noted that performance extends to sexual practices themselves. Women often "perform" or "fake" orgasm using their bodies and voices. My findings support the notion that women in short- and long-term relationships do performance work both within the sexual encounter itself and in relation to their wider social group. As Jolene, fifty-one, stated, "I've never enjoyed it [sex]. It's like something I'm supposed to do. Why? Because I'm a woman. And women are expected to. That's how you keep a guy happy. I'm such a good actress." As further evidence of performance work, Maria, twenty-two, is often preoccupied by the need to "tuck in her stomach" during sex. But Maria`s performance of normative heterosexuality apparently extends to her conversations with friends as well. She reflected, "I caught myself doing it so many times. Just pretending like when high school girls talk about sex. Like, it's so great and everything," adding, "I could tell that a lot of them … don't feel it was really good. It was just that they felt good about having sex and being able to say that they had good sex, but they didn't really." Contrary to Duncombe and Marsden (1996), Maria's account suggests that this type of outward performance or "deep acting" is not exclusive to long-term relationships, but is seen as a standard feature of teenage heterosexuality.

Performance work is a painful task for women with chronic genital pain. Susan, sixty-two, recalled the consequences of performing sexual enjoyment: "There were times when … I'd just go ahead and do it anyhow. And it would hurt a lot afterwards." Linda, twenty-six, who had been diagnosed with a sexual pain disorder, recalled "playing it off" or "sticking it out," pretending not to be in "excruciating" pain in order to have "penetration." She claimed she would "hide it from him [her partner]" because she "didn't want him to know he was hurting" her. She therefore "turned the lights out" and "cleaned up" before her partner could see the resulting "blood" from the "open wound" that would form as a result of these encounters. Participants who identified as having a medically defined sexual pain problem were not the only ones who claimed to be familiar with enduring pain in order to take part in intercourse. Faye, forty-two, described lack of sexual desire and arousal as her main sexual problems. She claimed she frequently had painful sex with former partners when she was not aroused, one time shortly after giving birth. She admitted, "I ignored the pain," an experience she remembered as being "amazingly painful."

Finally, many participants developed sexual-avoidance strategies, a form of work in and of itself. The techniques employed in such avoidance work included "falling asleep before he did" (Nicola) and "pretending to have my period for longer than I did" (Kate). Before getting divorced, Celia encouraged her husband to travel more often and made sure she was "busy doing laundry, cooking, cleaning" upon his return. There was general consensus that avoidance work was not a sustainable long-term strategy. Of the women quoted above as engaging in avoidance work, Nicola and Louise claimed their partners divorced them in part because of their strategies for avoiding sex. Elizabeth eventually opted for discipline work, and Kate, a firm believer in "faking it," juggled avoidance work with performance work as a means of sustaining her marriage.

## "Work with Me": Sex Experts and Sex Work

As in the case of authors of sexual self-help manuals, the practitioners I interviewed did not question the notion that successful heterosexuality should require "work," a tenet that informed their approach to treating women's sexual difficulties – indeed, all of them referred to the therapies they used with their clients or patients as "work." Consider the "work" metaphors in this account by this practitioner: "They do this *work* at home. Then if this is okay and they're not sure, I usually let them know when I think they can attempt intercourse. I usually say, 'I don't want you to have intercourse in the beginning when *we're working*.' Because all those things we're doing at the beginning for the pain cycle, if the penis goes in the vagina and causes pain, that's undoing what we've *worked towards*. So I usually let them know, 'Okay, I think you're getting ready for intercourse'" (emphasis added). The sex therapist referred to clients as taking part in sex work generally, or "couples work" and "singles work" specifically. One pelvic physiotherapist referred to her role as "working with them [women] … to reach sexual goals."

Pelvic physiotherapists described the exercises they prescribe using a "work/rest" metaphor. At one point during the interview, one practitioner pointed to a biofeedback readout, explaining that the flat lines represented "rest" or relaxation and the jagged lines "work" or the tightening of the pelvic floor muscles. She pointed to the lines on the readout, and stated, "This is rest-cycle, work-cycle, rest, work." At the end of this workout, the therapist said, the pelvic floor muscles are "fatigued" from the amount of work they have done. Both the pelvic physiotherapist and the sexual medicine specialist suggest women do their own work at home, which they actually referred to as "homework." Describing "homework," the specialist stated, "She's doing all this work on her own. That's mainly where all the work occurs. Not here in the office." Similarly, the pelvic physiotherapist commented, "I'm really a believer that … they need to be doing work at home, in-between our visits, in order for them to get better." The sex therapist, however, claimed not to be a fan of "homework," as she believed a professional should necessarily facilitate sex work.

Of all the types of sex work, the interview accounts suggest that discipline work is the option sex experts are most likely to advocate. Jackson and Scott (1997) have pointed to the inconsistency in messages from sex experts who frequently suggest that sex should be "spontaneous" even though they require "working harder and practicing in order to achieve the best possible outcome" (p. 562). Whether the practitioners I interviewed were employed in fields relating to mental or physical "health," they shared the goal of disciplining mental and physical sexual responses, but emphasized different aspects depending on their disciplinary background. The sex therapist privileged the *mental* disciplining of sexual response, often prescribing hypnosis. She stated: "I'm using it [hypnosis] to help people *feel more positive* because often people have a lot of *negative associations with sex*. Either they don't like it, *they don't find it arousing, it hurts*, whatever which of course, doesn't help for success of a good sexual experience" (emphasis added). Her basic strategy was to alter the woman's mental and physical reactions to certain types of sexual activity, rather than to alter social expectations of heterosexual sex. The other practitioners I interviewed use a more hands-on, desensitization approach dedicated to altering the physiological aspects of discipline work. As the pelvic physiotherapist explained: "We're doing a lot of *deprogramming* or *reprogramming* in this type of *work* so the [nerve] receptors learn that touch *does not mean pain*. So, if they start by using the little insert first and they're successful, it does a lot for them psychologically. They're doing a lot for the vaginal tissues, and they'll have to *relearn* that touch is okay. And *touch does not mean burning and stinging*. So, if they start with this and then gradually go up" (emphasis added).

In this psychological "deprogramming" and "reprogramming," women are taught to alter their response to normative sexual practices, rather than to redefine sexual practices and the expectations placed on them. When some were unwilling to do sex work, they were chastised by sexual advice professionals. For example, Charlene was told by her sex therapist that she "must" do "whatever it takes," "read books," "look at pictures," "use toys," "masturbate," even though, as she explained, she was "too tired" from her double shift of paid manual work and family care.

To a certain extent, sexual advice practitioners encouraged men to be "re-skilled" (Duncombe and Marsden, 1996) through discipline work. A number of practitioners whom participants in the study referred to required that male partners attend sessions. They further counselled men to take a more active approach to their partners' sexual difficulties. The sex therapist explained her views on the man's role in sex work by stating, "She may not have an orgasm because her partner doesn't have a clue how to stimulate her and he's taking two minutes of foreplay and moving on to intercourse. And so you want him there. You don't just want to be telling her." Women who accessed treatment from the sexual medicine centre were pleased to involve their partners. Only Charlene viewed this policy as "harsh," stating her centre physician was "furious" when her partner missed one appointment. This physician told her, "He should be here at all future appointments" because she had seen "too many relationships break up over it." In reality, it was often the women who were responsible for seeking and carrying out this work, and their partners were often the ones who encouraged them to do so in the first place. Samantha, twenty-four, said her partner "encouraged me to talk to my doctor." Louise's partner asked her, "Can you get your doctor to give you something so that you can get your sex drive back?" to which she responded, "Can you talk to your doctor and get him to give you something to stop yours?" Unable to understand Ruth's "inability to orgasm," her partner suggested she take part in this study as a form of sex work.

The practitioners I interviewed construed performance work as a normal, though not necessarily ideal, feature of heterosexual relationships, and they therefore did not advocate it. Basson's (2002d) female sexual response cycle is evidence of this outlook. Performing sexual acts that did not necessarily bring sexual pleasure, or "going along with it" to maintain a strong relationship, is considered a standard part of the labour of love. "We've all done it," one practitioner confided.

> I mean, it is different for men. I mean, men, especially young men are very reluctant to go ahead and be sexual if they're not feeling anything right then. They just don't feel sexually, whatever. They had sex this morning or they masturbated or whatever. They've got something on their mind, they're fed up about something, they're just not feeling very sexual right now ... Chances are very high that tomorrow they'll feel sexual and the next day and the next day ... Whereas [with] women, those kinds of sexual feelings are just so infrequent ... so, yeah, the expectation for the man is, if I want to be sexual then I have to feel like it beforehand. For women, it's just, well, you might not be feeling like it beforehand, but in a healthy relationship you'd be feeling emotionally close, and wanting to increase that intimacy, wanting to maybe feel better about yourself, more feminine, more relaxed, whatever.

At the heart of this statement is the notion that it is "normal" for women to *pretend* to be interested in sex in order for genuine desire to follow. Performance work is therefore normalized as part of a medical framework for understanding gender and sexuality.

The need for performance work is also taken for granted in many of the popular sex manuals I reviewed with Gupta (Gupta & Cacchioni, 2013). Kevin Leman (2003), author of *Sheet Music* (2000), a popular sex manual, encourages his readers to have sex for the sake of a desiring partner. He writes, "This means there may be times when you have sex out of mercy, obligation, or commitment and without any real desire. Yes, it may feel forced," but not to worry, "You're acting out of love. You're honoring your commitment. And that's a wonderful thing to do" (p. 203). Comfort and Quilliam (2009), authors of the latest edition of the *Joy of Sex*, write, "in an established relationship, always at least try to respond to seduction" (p. 102). Similarly, Chia, Chia, Abrams, and Abrams (2002) write, "if you or your partner is not interested in sex: Err in the direction of sex" (p. 180). Michelle Weiner Davis (2003) is a firm believer in what she terms "Nike Sex," or "just doing it," and she advises partners to relate to sex as a gift when it is offered. She claims that both pieces of advice (to give sex as a gift and to accept it) are "gender neutral"; sometimes the wife is the "low desire spouse" and the husband is the "high desire spouse," sometimes this pattern reversed. In writing about "Nike Sex," however, she also references Basson's (2002d) model of female sexual response, inferring that the low-desire spouse likely would be female.

The practitioners I interviewed discouraged avoidance work entirely, apparently because of its perceived non-sustainability. It was clear, however, that their client base, income, and job security depend on a market of women willing to engage in discipline work. All three sexual advice professionals I interviewed prioritized "keeping the couple together." When Olivia told her psychologist that she and her husband avoided "working on" or "dealing with" the issue that their marriage was "unconsummated," she was told, "Go to therapy and come back." The suggestion, therefore, was that mainly (mental) discipline work – changing the mental response to penetrative sex – would be necessary. She explained how she felt *before* hearing these comments: "At that time I was really proud of myself because I was following my choices. And that's just not right for me right now. So that's fine. I was fine with it. It didn't bother me."

**Sex Work versus Sexual Pharmaceuticals**

If sex work is a "chore" for some women and enjoyable for others, how does the option of taking a sexual pharmaceutical measure up as an alternative? It seems that no sexual enhancement drug for women could possibly replace some of the well-liked discipline work strategies, particularly those that women with chronic genital pain engage in. Several participants highlighted the wish to "keep it natural," which they interpreted as not taking medication. Even if evidence of "the labour of love" ultimately confirms Tiefer's (1995) maxim that "sex is not a natural act," it is interesting that participants were attached to the notion of keeping sex "natural."

Following her empirical study of women's perceptions of experiences of menopause, Bransen (1992) noted a growing "natural genre" in interview accounts wherein "the dominant attitude" was "I would prefer to keep it natural" (p. 107). As evidence of this discourse, Amy, a physiotherapist, considered even lubricant gel to be an "unnatural" solution to vaginal dryness, stating, "I just don't like adding anything not natural to my sex life." Although the women in my study with sexual pain were enthusiastic about drugs to manage pain and their potential to enable intercourse, only three claimed they would be excited to try a sexual pharmaceutical drug for desire, arousal, and orgasm. Lauren, a university student, proclaimed, "I think there's something that should be a more natural solution to it and a more permanent solution ... people become dependent on it." Zoe, a radio documentary maker, stated bluntly, "I don't take pharmaceuticals." Celia, a nurse, was "ticked" (angry) when her GP offered her estrogen cream for vaginal dryness, stating, "She could have asked me if I was sexually active," which she had not been "for nine years." Grace, a cruise consultant, was initially pleased to be prescribed hormone replacement therapy cream for vaginal dryness, but she said she felt "angry," as evidence from clinical trials had since proven it to be "dangerous." By prescribing the cream, the doctor made her feel as though she was "biologically doomed" and that her "sexual days were over." Leanne, a scientist, did not view the testosterone cream she was prescribed off-label by her doctor as a panacea. She was concerned about "the long-term effects of taking testosterone, even in small doses," and stated, "I don't want to be on medication unless I have to be." She has since stopped taking testosterone, and has tried again to solve her inability to orgasm "naturally." Louise, an office manager, refused clinical counselling when the psychiatrist told her, "Well, if you're not going to take medication, I won't see you," even though she was pregnant with her second child. Judging by comments made by the women in my study, a "pink" Viagra would not appeal to everyone.

## Conclusions

As detailed in a myriad studies mapping women's domestic, beauty, body, and emotional labour, meeting exacting standards of successful heterosexuality is "hard work," especially for women. Why should heterosexual sexual practices require anything less? Discussing this kind of work challenges heterosexual romantic and/or essentialist discourses in which sex is indeed seen as a "natural" act. It is clear from my findings that sex work is advocated in the context not only of self-help, but also of clinical and/or professional, face-to-face therapies and treatments. The sex experts who advocated discipline work, and warned against performance or avoidance work, had an undeniable financial interest in doing so.

Heterosexual women who cannot or will not mirror the expected norms of heterosex seem to be particularly targeted or compelled to do the work of heterosexual improvement. Throwing in the towel on this kind of work is seen as an apathetic and dangerous strategy for relationship longevity. Women in long-term relationships who are unable or unwilling to engage in penis-vagina intercourse are see particularly as risking their relationships if they do not make an effort to reprogram. Although Duncombe and Marsden (1996) suggested this trend was unique to couples only at a certain stage in their relationship, my findings suggest that single women without sexual partners or with short-term sexual partners engage in sex work, too. Indeed, there is now a vast market of medicalized and non-medicalized approaches to working on sex. Whereas some approaches focus on disciplining or "programming" the mind or body towards the standard heterosexual script, increasingly even medical experts advocate mental *and* physical discipline for ultimate success. Although performance and avoidance work are common strategies for dealing with the pressures of normative sex, the sexual advice practitioners I interviewed warned against them.

Of course, men take part in relationship-based sex work as well, but even while the face of hegemonic masculinity is evolving and changing, men do not seem to be as involved in the "project of the self" (Giddens, 1991) to the same degree as women, with regards to self-improvement generally and sexual improvement specifically. Part of the reason for this might be gender socialization, the historical sexual division of "emotional" labour (Hochschild, 1983), and the way that the post–sexual revolution self-help industry has explicitly targeted women just as they began to experience greater sexual freedom (Erenreich & English, 1978; Hawkes, 1996; Jeffries, 1990). Now that capacity for sexual enjoyment is an integral part of women's sexual capital, the stakes are particularly high.

Whether sex work is seen as a chore or enjoyable, my research suggests that certain forms of sex work seem to offer some kind of process that cannot be replaced by simply popping a pill. Although my findings are minimal with regards to women's attitudes to the notion of sexual pharmaceuticals, the informants' sentiments might be seen as part of a wider backlash against this example of the medicalization of everyday life.

# 5 Refusing Heteronormative Sex Work

To enjoy or not to enjoy the labour of love? Are these the only options? There are, of course, alternatives to working on improving the performance and enactment of normative sex. Rather than working towards mastering, strategically mimicking, or carefully avoiding sexual practices, at some point in their lives one-third of the women in this study made changes to their sexual relationships and activities and/or to the value they placed on them. Refusing sex work involved challenging normative definitions of sex and even the overall importance of sexual activity. What might be thought of as "queering" the heteronormative script by which sexual function and dysfunction are judged might involve prioritizing sexual acts typically categorized as foreplay or valuing non-goal-oriented masturbation (not necessarily ending in orgasm) as acceptable sexual activity on a par with intercourse. Another way of refusing to work on sexual improvement was seen in the stories of participants who deprioritized sex all together. Although none took on the identity of "asexuality" as reflected in the small but growing self-proclaimed grassroots movement I discuss later in the chapter, some of the participants questioned the overall importance placed on sexual relationships, institutions, and practices. For these women, such strategies tended to represent a change in sexual practice, rather than a shift in overall identity. Regardless, some felt restricted when making sexual choices for financial reasons, and some bore material costs as a result of their decision to refuse the labour of love.

## Queering Normative Heterosex

Whether it is possible to "queer" heterosex and what the implications might be of doing so have been the subject of debate in feminist and queer theory. Much of this debate centres on the possibility of queering heterosexual identity – that is, becoming a queer-identified heterosexual (Schlichter, 2004). But as queer theorists such as Judith Butler (1990) emphasize, the very notion of "queer" resists the stability demanded by identity categories.[1] Halperin (1995), for instance, argues that "queer" does not refer to a determinate object. Rather, as Burrill (2009) states, "queer is by definition *whatever* is at odds with the normal, the legitimate, the dominant. *There is nothing in particular to which it necessarily refers.* It is an identity without an essence" (p. 62; emphasis added). Queer might be better understood as a position, rather than an identity – one that might shift with times, norms, and expectations.

The question of whether heterosexual sexual *practices* can be queered and what the implications of this might be is linked to a slightly different debate. Since the so-called sexual revolution and the rise of second-wave feminism, various attempts have been made to challenge firmly entrenched phallocentric notions of heterosex. Radical feminists in the 1970s and 1980s sought to politicize and deprioritize penetration as a strategy for reconstituting heterosexuality as an institution (Dworkin, 1987; Jeffreys, 1990). Using the tools of deconstruction, post-structuralist feminists in the 1990s attempted to "wrench penetration out of the heterosexual matrix" (Smart, 1996) as a way of destabilizing its meaning, power, and privilege. These efforts were also part and parcel of a post–"sex war," "sex positive" movement to make room for a feminist discourse on penetrative pleasure, whether by penis, finger, fist, or object. During the same decade, Cobb (1997) and others began to advocate for the promotion of heterosexual "outercourse," a term conveyed within the lexicon of safe sex advice related to sexually transmitted infection and teen pregnancy prevention.

More recently, however, Thomas (2000) and O'Rourke (2005) have discussed the emergence of a "straight-queer" who "celebrates non-normative heterosexualities, the queer practices of straights, and the lives and loves of those men and women who choose to situate themselves beyond the charmed circle at the heteronormative centre" (O'Rourke, 2005, p. 112). By this definition, it seems that the project of *queering* heterosex is more inclusive than the radical feminist project, moves beyond the strict focus on discourse as seen in the post-structuralist emphasis, and is more politicized than the neoliberal public health promotion of "outercourse" (Cobb, 1997). Speaking to the challenges and potentials of a broad conceptualization of queer, Elia (2003) argues that we must call on individuals to be "architects of their own relationship construction, while at the same time employing the most rigorous self-reflexivity so as to avoid various and sundry manifestations of elitism, prejudice, and oppression that are byproducts of sex and relationship hierarchies" (p. 78). O'Rourke (2005) is hopeful of a new, inclusive, queer practice that "embraces all straight men, straight women, gay men, lesbians, bisexuals, the transgendered, transsexuals, the intersexed, and gives them the right" (p. 114), as Segal (1994) states, to "fuck if, when, how, and as they choose."

Having conducted an ethnography of women who experience pelvic pain, Labuski (2014) argues, however, that such statements "do not fully capture the specificity – nor the social and sexual significance – of being physically unable to participate in an activity by which one's own sexual orientation is almost completely defined" (p. 311) – in other words, what Kaler (2006) refers to as the "paradigmatic heterosexual act" (p. 51) of penis-vagina intercourse. Indeed, although several of the participants in this study challenged the heteronormative script, rarely did they make this challenge from the ontological and political stance that theorists such as O'Rourke (2005) conjure when describing the "straight-queer." Perhaps the distinction Beasley et al. (2012) make between the politics of sexual "transgression" and those of "subversion" is a useful intervention in this discussion: sex might be transgressed non-deliberately, or it might be subverted, meaning a "reflexive undermining of heteronormativity that can produce challenges to or shifts in the norm" (p. 5).

The participants' refusal to work towards (particularly hetero) sexual norms can be characterized mainly as transgressive, more than subversive. Three of the women who "queered" heterosex did so mainly after first exhausting sex work techniques, and then, in some cases, after a professional had suggested changing sexual scripts and expectations as an alternative – perhaps as a "last resort." A number of sex advice practitioners make challenging normative sexuality central to their approach (for example, Hall, 2001; Kleinplatz, 2012; Ogden, 2001). Although none of the practitioners I interviewed or whom participants described was an explicit example of this approach, a minority advocated a shift in thinking about or doing heterosexuality. For instance, Danielle, the forty-four-year-old teacher who once viewed herself as an "android" for her inability to have intercourse, referred to one sexual medicine specialist she consulted as "different from all the other doctors I saw." According to Danielle, this physician was the first expert to ask her, "What sort of sexual activities can you do that are mutually satisfying and … not intercourse?" Danielle elaborated on the influence of this physician on her views: "All of a sudden, it just came together at the same time where I said, 'You know what? I've got to stop thinking about this. I have to. I just have to. I have to change my mindset'." She claimed, "I'm not feeling like an android anymore. I am very much in love with [my partner], as he is with me. We're very happy. We have a good, good life."

Samantha, a twenty-four-year-old actor, claimed never to have had an orgasm despite the efforts of her "eager-to-please," long-term partner. She consulted a sexual medicine specialist, who told her, "It's something that will happen. Just don't let it become a big focal point in your life." According to Samantha, this advice led her and her partner to "try some different things" in the realm of "foreplay" that "felt really good." As a result, she claimed she was "not really distressed about" her inability to orgasm. Indicative of the remarkably more upbeat attitudes of those who had queered sex, rather than doing sex work, she reflected:

> I guess, for me, in terms of sexual experiences, my boyfriend and I still have a lot of fun. It still feels very good. We feel very close. It's a good close, together type feeling. And I think I probably value that a lot more, and that's what I've always pictured sexuality as. More than just the orgasm. But I feel like I'm getting a good 80–90 per cent of what I want. It's just this one small thing that I'm missing. And I'd really like it. It would be great if I could have it, but at the same time I'm fulfilled in so many other ways that it's not … taking over.

Samantha might count herself as missing 10–20 per cent of a normative sexual experience, but she nonetheless claimed to feel "fulfilled in so many other ways." Monica readjusted her view of sex to fit her inability to orgasm through studying and practising Kundalini yoga. About this approach, she explained, "You're educated in a way where you embody more the wholeness of sexuality, understanding, not focusing only on sex and having to have the orgasm or the fornicating impact." She claimed to prioritize: "Just being able to be alive within your own being and connecting with your own sexuality. Yeah, just for you to have that awareness to understand. I think … people [would] not [be] so consumed with the pressures to have [an] orgasm. Not just focus on that one thing … It's not just that one goal to have the orgasm, but it's just connecting with your sensuality and all your senses." Although this comment could be constructed as setting up a particular sexual framework in its own right, Monica highlighted a variety of sensory experiences other than orgasm and even referred to her lack of orgasms as "not a big deal."

Zoe, a documentary film maker in her twenties, stands out as somewhat more subversive in her approach. She allowed herself to explore a range of sexualities that fall outside what Rubin (1984) termed the "charmed circle" of normative sex, and she was more reflexive about the process. From early heterosex onwards, Zoe felt she had problems with desire, arousal, and orgasm. She first entered a sexual relationship with her current partner when she was eighteen. As she explained, "My interest would peak when we would stumble across something interesting, but then that would always make him feel uncomfortable, so then he'd shut down." After seven years of a monogamous partnership, she had "an affair." After ending the affair, which had enabled her to experiment with an expansion of her sexual repertoire, Zoe broke up with her long-time partner and "explored my sexuality in terms of my bisexuality" with a queer-identified female. However, she described this relationship as "very frustrating," and a "total repeat situation of [her male partner] again," as lack of communication seemed to play a role in the dwindling of their sexual pleasure. Although she claimed that her sex life did not improve directly through this relationship, she attributed her "involvement with the Queer community," and her friendships with people "who were much more open about sex," as leading her to change her previously narrow views of sex. She was inspired to experiment with masturbating, an activity she formerly thought "only men do," an experience she described as a "turning point," stating, "It did feel really good to be able to take care of my sexual needs." Later, she and her former male partner got back together, which one might read as heterosexuality's reinstating itself. She described the heterosex they practised going forward, however, as somehow different in that "incarnation of their relationship," as she termed it. According to Zoe, when she and her partner got involved in "the rave scene" or "the party scene," which she described as characterized by gender and sexual experimentation, they began to share a more "fluid" outlook on what sex might entail. She reflected: "The party scene kind of changed [her partner's views on sex] ... a little bit. I'm not sure entirely in what way. I think because when it started ... in the party scene, it opened up a lot. In the early days of the party scene, gender was really fluid. You know, girls wore pants, boys would wear pink. There was just a really neat flow there. I think that opened him up a lot. That was interesting." She described the way that this "flow," or "opening up," reshaped their sex lives together: "We brought a lot of play into it. Like a lot of dress-up boots and high heels and things like that that we never really felt comfortable with before, [things] we'd kind of explored in the first incarnation of our relationship, but every time we'd touched it, we left it."

The above examples illustrate instances of changing sexual expectations and scripts, prioritizing the most straightforward means to sexual enjoyment over sexual "normality." The participants in my study came to this alternative approach through medicalized and non-medicalized paths. In every case, when describing this shift, they sounded more upbeat or positive. It is impossible to know, however, if the positive framing of these shifts was simply a reverse discourse, a new norm for those with sexual difficulties, or a forced happy ending to a tale of distress and perceived dysfunction. One could also argue that the changing of a mindset about the normative sexual script is yet another form of discipline work. Therefore, I offer these findings of queering the heterosexual script optimistically, but cautiously.

## Exiting Heterosexual Relationships and Prioritizing the Non-sexual

A movement has emerged among young people in the West to challenge the notion that one must be sexual. Representative of the "asexual movement," the Asexual Visibility and Education Network (AVEN) is an international, grassroots network that positions itself as separate from abstinence movements like the US-based, Christian fundamentalist "Silver Ring Thing," associated with religious reactions to the liberalization of sex and the AIDS pandemic. According to the AVEN website,[2] "Celibate people choose to abstain from sexual relationships, while asexual people simply don't feel compelled to conform to them." A key tenet of asexuality as an identity is that non-sexual relationships are equally as important as sexual relationships that are seen as being imbued with greater value. AVEN explains, "Non-sexual relationships can be just as close as sexual ones. Sexuality is one way to express emotion in a close relationship, but it is by no means THE way. Anything that can be done through sexuality (emotional expression, fun, physical closeness, etc.) can be done nonsexually." AVEN defines an asexual person simply as "a person who does not experience sexual attraction," and explains that there are a huge number of practices associated with this identity. According to AVEN, some asexual people have romantic,

non-physical relationships, while others do not. Within romantic relationships, some asexual-identified people engage in "sexual" activities as a way of expressing affection or pleasing their partners, others
do not. Some asexual people masturbate, many do not. AVEN distin-
guishes between asexual and sexual masturbation by explaining that
the former is about physical release and sometimes fantasy, but does
not lead to the wish to have interactive sexual contact with another
person.

Non-sexual intimate relationships have long been the interest of feminist scholars (see, for example, Smith-Rosenberg, 1975;). In an exploration of the cartography of asexuality's "pre-history," Przybylo (2013)
notes that mid-twentieth-century sexual orientation models often
took asexuality as a normal, yet neglected point on a sexual continuum. Whereas Kinsey, Pomeroy, and Martin's (1948) seven-point scale
assumed some level of sexuality in each individual, the work of Storms
(1979) and Nurius (1983) "took for granted the notion that asexuality
must exist" (Przybylo, 2013, p. 227). By contrast, in their emphasis on
normalizing sexual pleasure, Masters, Johnson, and Kolodny (1986)
associated asexuality with negative psychological traits. Recently, however, on the tail of the asexuality movement, contemporary scholars
such as Bogaert (2004), Brotto and colleagues (Brotto et al., 2010; Brotto &
Yule, 2011), and Prause and Graham (2007), working from a psychology model, have attempted to legitimize asexuality using empirical
strategies.

The asexuality movement flies in the face of the notion that a lack of
sexual urges and abilities signals "dysfunction" that must be worked
on and overcome. As a key player in the institutionalization of female
sexual dysfunction, Laura Berman has been vocal about her scepticism regarding the veracity of claims by asexuals. On her Oprah Radio
talk show, she hosted a program titled "Is Asexuality Real?" (Berman,
2010a). In a baffled tone, she vented, "This just really kind of annoys
me. And listen, you know me ... I try to be *really* open minded ... There's
this website, asexuality.org, and there's this whole community of asexuals ... [W]hat they say is that an asexual is someone who does not
experience sexual attraction, unlike celibacy [where one might feel sexual but suppress this feeling]". She later explained what it is about the
asexual identity and lifestyle that she questions as a sex therapist. First,
the asexual identity is complicated for her because it resists stability. In
an accusatory voice, she commented on the "considerable amount of

diversity in the asexual community ... [T]hey talk about how you can have attraction ... you can masturbate ... you can have romantic relationships ... so what makes you an asexual?" Second, asexuality flies in the face of a pathological model of sexual dysfunction. Laura Berman is convinced that there must be an underlying cause or etiology of this lack of prioritization of the sexual. She questioned:

> Why aren't you acting on sex? Is that you are kind of skeeved out by sex? ... [W]hat is it? Is it just that you have a low libido ... ? And why do you need an asexual community? ... Why not just say you're turned off by the idea of sex. Why not just say, "Something happened to me when I was young." Or "I'm just freaked out of the idea of sex." Or "I don't want to have sex." ... But if you're still experiencing a certain degree of desire, attraction, you have a certain sexual orientation ... And *it is* by choice because ... you are choosing not have sex ... They say ... that they're attracted to a particular gender and that they get aroused, but it's just not associated with a desire to find a sexual partner or partners ... asexual people generally don't see their lack of sexuality as a problem to be corrected ... I don't know ... we'll have to explore that.

It seems that the discourse on asexuality threatens the coherence of the medical framework in which a certain level of sexual desire is the norm, from which any aberration signals a psychological or physiological problem that likely should be addressed through expert intervention.

By contrast Marny Hall (2001), a New View supporter and former specialist in lesbian sex therapy, reflecting on her thirty years of experience of counselling women who deemed themselves as experiencing "lesbian bed death,"[3] came to the following realization: "[M]y prescriptions for a healthy sex life, despite the lesbian-friendly window dressing I had given it, were laced with the phallocentric values and suppositions that I had imbibed as a trainee. Now that lesbian bed death seemed a particularly oppressive fiction, a 'condition' to be deconstructed rather than treated, I could no longer, in good conscience, be a lesbian sex therapist. Instead, I became an anti-sex therapist" (p. 168). The notion of "anti-sex therapy" is timely. Hall's approach to this model is to offer education on alternatives to those who do not feel or want to be particularly sexual, advocating against stigma and pathology.

Although none of the participants in my study readily identified as embracing an "asexual" identity as expressed by the burgeoning "asexual movement," some challenged normative heterosexuality by prioritizing non-sexual aspects of life and non-sexual relationships. Among these participants, women in their twenties and thirties talked about prioritizing non-sexual relationships and activities as a temporary strategy. For Jas, twenty-seven, the most effective way of dealing with sexual difficulties was "taking a vacation from men." During her early twenties, Jas felt that she "was not able to conduct any sort of healthy relationship with a guy," and did not understand why people "thought sex was enjoyable." She explained, "Even if I wanted to or not, if somebody wanted to have sex with me, I would just very easily comply because I didn't know how to say … I didn't know my voice to say 'no'." Despite consulting friends and her general practitioner and receiving counselling therapy for her sexual problems, Jas felt she was unable to break a pattern of having unwanted, non-pleasurable sex. She referred to her pause from heterosex as "my turning point," when she began "suddenly seeing myself from a different perspective. Like, I stepped outside of myself and said, 'What are you doing?'" Jas never approached her sojourn from sexual relationships as a long-term strategy. But she described this "vacation" period as "healing within myself" and as instrumental to her ability to engage in pleasurable sex again.

Similarly, Maria, a twenty-two-year-old participant with "orgasm issues" who had sought no professional advice, used '"taking a break" from sexual relationships as a short-term strategy for dealing with these issues. As Maria explained, "After my third relationship, I was single. I didn't want relationships. I hated them. So, I was single for three years." During this time, through personal reflection, rather than any expert advice, she decided that she wanted to find a "more experienced" and even "more mature" sexual partner. She stated, "I guess I [had] to learn to say, 'You know, I don't feel like having sex tonight.' Or 'Can we do this instead?' And I guess that goes with finding a better partner."

In this study, middle-aged participants who refused sex work seemed to adopt the non-sexual approach as a long-term strategy. Celia, a fifty-six-year-old nurse, said she had never enjoyed sexual activity. Rather than seek professional advice, however, she chose a divorce. She described her single, non-sexual life as analogous to "finding myself," which "was important to me." Aside from dreading sex with her husband due to lack of interest, arousal, *and* orgasm, Celia explained that, in her marriage, she was "sort of losing myself."

She described her divorce as "very liberating," and elaborated on the divorce process:

> And he tried to control me even beyond the separation agreement by saying, "Let's look for some place for you to live." "No, I'm going to look." Then we'd go in the car and he say, "That house isn't too far from us. That will work for the kids." "No I don't want a house. Then I'll have to maintain it." And when I did find a house that is suitable, he asked if he could look over the purchaser agreement so he could help me. And I go, "No! This is *mine*." And there was another incident where I was dropping the kids off and I gave him a ride in my new car, which was a used car but I'd sold the station wagon he got me and got me a Honda ... I could see him looking at me quite differently, like, "You bought a car on your own. You bought a condo on your own." And it just felt very liberating. And then he sort of gave me a little bit more space. Maybe a bit more respect.

Although Celia expressed that she was lonely from time to time, having not met another long-term companion, she was content with her newfound freedom. She claimed she was now looking for a companion who would be similarly willing to prioritize non-sexual aspects of the relationship, someone "who will make me flush when he did something non-sexual that really endeared me to him."

Similarly, Hannah, a fifty-three-year-old single mother who recently returned to university to do post-graduate work, divorced her partner, with whom she did not enjoy sex. She described this decision and her subsequent relocation from a small town to Vancouver as "self-empowerment for me." She elaborated, "I feel my own strength." Hannah was now interested in finding a good friend whom she could "go to a concert with" or "go for a ride" with, "but not romance." Since "swearing off men," another participant, Jolene, missed physical affection, but did not miss penetrative sex. She mused, "do I miss sex itself, the act? No. Do I miss the hugging and holding? Yes, supposing it's there. Not hop on, hop off like a jack rabbit."

Nicola, a thirty-four-year-old school teacher, was the only participant to take the non-sexual route by finding a companion who similarly wanted a non-sexual long-term relationship. Describing herself as having "low sexual desire," Nicola was married for ten years to her "high school sweetheart," a man she described as "different sexually." Initially, she attempted to fake it and avoid sex to deal with the imbalance between his "high sex drive" and her "low sex drive," stating,

"I had sex when I didn't want to. And then that hatred grew." Her marriage ended with him leaving her, "and then … my life really changed. I mean, it changed for the better." After a few years of single life, Nicola met her current long-term partner, who, she said, "doesn't need to be sexual with me or to be sexual to get satisfaction." She claimed that her new partner defies the notion that all men have a "high sex drive." Reflecting on her current partnership, she said, "I'm really not a very sexual person but [now] I don't feel guilt for it. I don't feel like I'm not doing my duty … It's completely different."

Although I have attempted to show that it is possible for women to deprioritize sexual activity and relationships, even if they do not take on an asexual identity per se, Labuski (2014) is slightly more pessimistic about what she terms "behavioural asexuality" among heterosexual-identified women. There might be an overlap in experience between heterosexual-identified "behavioural asexuals" and those who identify as asexual, but Labuski cautions against conflating the two: "There are notable distinctions between choosing to (temporarily) abstain from intercourse (and/or to frame other behaviours as less than or non-sexual) and being corporeally compelled to make those same adjustments" (p. 310). In her view, when women with genital pain make this choice, they "circumvent episodes of painful sex," but "close off other possibilities as well: both non-penetrative sexual activity and a more fully affirmed asexual identity and lifestyle" (p. 311).

## Refusing Sex Work: The Role of Material Factors

Since the 1990s theorists have imagined a contemporary sexual landscape of "sexual postmodernization" (Simon, 1996) that celebrates "process, paradox, and play" (Tyler, 2004), or what Giddens (1992) refers to as the "pure relationship," characterized by "equality and emotional give and take" (p. 58) and "plastic sexuality" – that is, sex for pleasure's sake. And yet, as Jackson (1999) argues, structural and material factors continue to underlie the sense of choices and options that women perceive as having when it comes to sex. She warns that "discourses do not float free from material structures or material inequalities characterizing the societies in which they are produced" (p. 181). Duncombe and Marsden (1996) similarly emphasize material factors, stating, "[interpersonal] sex work takes place in the context of an interpersonal balance of power … Undoubtedly, the balance of power in such exchanges tends to be tilted toward men" (p. 222).

The heterosexual participants in my study who were financially dependent on their partners were less likely to refuse to work on the achievement of heterosexual norms. From their perspective, the material "costs" outweighed the "benefits" that might be gained from having greater freedom to express themselves sexually. For example, Kate, a forty-three-year-old mother without post-secondary education, career training, or a paid job, rationalized doing sex work as part of her duty to her family. She stated: "It's worth it for [my husband]. Yeah, I think it's working where my daughter has two parents, where my husband is not wound up, and I'm just doing something that I don't find very pleasant and would like to find a lot more pleasant … I'm well aware that I love my husband and I want to stay with my husband. Our life is great. It's almost like … you don't want to do many things but you do them. So, I have sex probably twice a week."

Indeed, refusing the labour of love roused fears of financial insecurity, especially among participants with children and/or those who did not have paid careers of their own. As employed women without children, queering heterosex or deprioritizing sexual activity was an easier choice for Jas, Maria, Danielle, Samantha, and Nicola. By contrast, as mothers with less financial independence, Jolene, Celia, and Hannah bore clear financial costs from their decision to challenge the norms of heterosexuality. Jolene, who lives below the poverty line, was aware that her decision to forsake sexual relationships and live as a single mother placed her in a vulnerable position. She explained, "Right now, I exist day to day by just being able to put a roof over my head, feed myself." Celia reflected on her decision to divorce, stating, "I didn't know financially how I would handle it … I was so emotionally in need of getting away, I was ready to go with nothing, meaning no money and no nothing. I would beg, borrow, and steal, but I wouldn't take anything from him, which was not too bright … So, [custody] was half time with me and half with him, and there was no exchange of support even though he made a heck of a lot more money than me. I did not want it. Actually, that turned out to be financially quite hard." Celia, like many women in her situation, despite having performed all the unpaid labour involved in her heterosexual relationship, including child rearing, did not feel entitled to a divorce settlement. Another participant, Hannah, decided to file for divorce after years of emotional and physical abuse, and although she has raised her ex-partner's children, one of whom is disabled and requires full-time care, she did "not receive any child support anymore – nothing." She is now disputing this legal issue in court.

## Conclusions

A number of sexual identities and practices present a challenge to narrow definitions of "real" and pleasurable sex as necessarily involving foreplay followed by coitus followed by orgasm. Aside from the very small sample of lesbian and bisexual participants in my study, the majority remained firmly entrenched in a heterosexual identity. About one-third, however, challenged heteronormativity to some extent by refusing or giving up on normative sex work. Some did so by forgoing the heteronormative script, others by breaking free of heterosexual relationships and institutions such as marriage. In many ways, their actions were more transgressive than subversive. Nevertheless, it is remarkable that these women, on the whole, sounded more upbeat and positive than the women who engaged in the work of improving their sexual functioning.

As Jackson (1999) claims, "Our capacity to undo gender and heterosexuality is constrained by the structural inequalities which sustain them" (p. 181). Material factors proved influential in women's decision to take part in sex work as well as in guiding the level of ease with which they were able to make changes to the status quo of their sexual scripts and/or the priority they placed on sex. Particularly for women with children and no paid career, financial considerations were central to their decision to perform sex work. Even still, some participants in these circumstances boldly chose to challenge what has long been conceived of simply as "a labour of love."

# 6 A Woman's Work Is Never Done

Contrary to the drug industry and the medics it funds, sexual "short-comings" have not been eliminated by providing men a blue pill and women a pink one. The pseudo-feminist, neoliberal rhetoric of "choice" and individual "empowerment" that forms the basis of industry hype over the search for a sexual pharmaceutical for women is problematic on several levels. The motivation behind efforts to find such a drug is profit, not pleasure. In clinical trials of sexual dysfunction drugs, increasingly vague and subjective endpoints are used to measure efficacy and a consistently high placebo effect is downplayed. The speed at which key opinion leaders are willing to change their public statements on sexual dysfunction based on which drug they have been paid to promote is telling. Even when a drug is found to carry serious side effects, as is the case with Viagra, the risks are minimized by the maker and by the medical spokespeople hired to promote it.

As Leonore Tiefer and other New View supporters argue, understanding sexual problems as simply the result of poor blood flow, hormonal imbalance, or the short-circuiting of neurological hardwiring ignores key social, economic, and political factors that shape sexual pleasure and displeasure. Some sexual medicine physicians, such as Rosemary Basson (2001a, 2001b, 2001c, 2002), highlight numerous personal and interpersonal motivations for wanting to engage in sexual activity. But Tiefer emphasizes wider socio-political factors and argues that, in any event, sex is "more like dancing than digestion."

I started this book by mapping the polemic that has emerged in the sexual pharmaceutical era, and by arguing in support of the doubts that have been raised about the promise of these drugs to transform women's sex lives. However, I wanted to intervene in these debates by putting the question of sexual pharmaceuticals aside and asking women who define themselves as having sexual problems how they understood these issues and what they did to solve them in everyday life. I also wanted to understand better how low- and high-tech ways of addressing sexual problems compared and/or depended on one another, and what all of this might tell us about medicalization and heteronormativity. Through my empirical analysis, I have drawn several conclusions about the supremacy and disruption of both medicalization and normative (especially hetero) sex. I also found that these two social processes are intimately linked in a reciprocal way.

Heterosexual women, particularly those with the means to afford it, have long engaged in a number of disciplinary body and beauty practices. Increasingly, the use of pharmaceuticals – from oral contraceptives for the treatment of acne to hormone replacement therapy for menopause and age-related symptoms – is part of the roster of celebrated gender conformity and heterosex in North America. It is easy to assume that a sexual pharmaceutical could be the next commercial product to add to this array of interventions shaping the appearance, youthfulness, and social acceptability of the gender-conforming, feminine, heterosexual subject. But even without an available sexual pharmaceutical drug, the women I interviewed for this study, from a range of age, racial, ethnic, national, and social class backgrounds, judged their sexuality in relation to very specific heterosexual norms, and felt compelled to analyse, monitor, and manage their and their partner's sexual experiences accordingly. Although some enjoyed honing their sexual talents, others felt it was a chore and/or part of a wider scheme of heterosexual coercion. Some also deemed the work of sexual improvement uncomfortable, unpleasant, and expensive. Discussions about women who experience sexual pain have been largely absent in feminist critiques of "female sexual dysfunction," But the women with this experience were the most distressed about their sexual problems of all the participants in my study, and for good reason: they faced the most sanctions as a result of their sexual difficulties.

Thus, despite wider pressures, some participants transgressed and perhaps even subverted the heteronormative framework, deciding to define what worked for them, rather than working on what did not. Others opted out of sexual activity and relationships all together because they wanted to, were advised to, or had no other options for a variety of reasons. The extent to which changing or forgoing celebrated sexual scripts represents a true challenge to the institution of heterosexuality remains to be seen. Given the material consequences these women faced as a result of their transgressions, the institution seemed at least threatened by their actions, while simultaneously reinforced.

## Understanding Sexual Problems: Through a Heteronormative Lens

Although there now might be more acceptance of women's active sexuality, this shift has been accompanied by new sexual pressures, anxieties, and rules that have particular consequences for those with inactive or difficult sexualities. The heterosexual women I interviewed for this book by and large judged their sexual problems in relation to a very narrow equation of successful sex as frequent foreplay, followed by coitus, ending in orgasm. In keeping with the existing sociological literature, these women confronted varying degrees of sexual coercion at a young age (Holland et al. 1998; Thompson 1990, 1995; Tolman, 2001) and in adult heterosexual relationships (Gavey, 1993, 2005; Jackson, 1999; Jackson & Scott, 1997). Contrary to the neoliberal, "post-feminist masquerade" (McRobbie, 2006) of sexual choice, empowerment, and freedom, a number of participants pointed to mental, physical, and sexual violence as major pressures informing their perceptions. Far from being unwitting dupes of male privilege, the majority of the women in this study actively resented these narrow views of sex.

Heterosexual-identified participants were aware that *the* essential ingredient for what is considered to be "real" sex is intercourse. Confirming Kaler's (2006) argument that women who are unable "to perform this one hallowed heterosexual activity … invoke images of gender failures, of women who were not really women" (p. 51), failing to meet this key heterosexual criteria led some to question their ontological sense of being "a woman." Many were unable to sustain their relationships for this very reason, while others in relationships lived in fear of "getting dumped" or of not meeting someone in the first place. Thus, it makes sense that the heterosexual-indentified women with chronic genital pain in this study understood their sexual problems in the most negative terms, faced the most interpersonal and social consequences for their sexual difficulties, and were the most positive about biomedical solutions. It is possible that even invasive and expensive band-aid solutions such as Botox for vaginismus will be attractive to women who can afford these technologies. Even if a woman has the will to engage in heterosexual intercourse, an incapacity to engage in heteronormative acts can easily compromise her sexual capital.

The study included only a very small sample of lesbian and bisexual participants. From their accounts, it seems that being involved in a same-sex relationship did not of itself seem to dissolve the pressures and influence of normative heterosexuality. As the existing literature suggests (see, for example, Jackson, 1999; Richardson, 1996), in many ways, these women still negotiated expectations associated with normative heterosexuality even though penis-vagina penetration was not central to their sexual repertoire.

Despite acute, bitter awareness of the norms of (particularly hetero) sex, some participants seem to have transgressed and even subverted these norms at various points. There was a remarkably more positive tone when informants described their decision to give up trying to be "normal" and focus instead on what could be pleasurable for them – a common sentiment among those who had refused sex work was that they were happier. Others deprioritized sexual activity and relationships in the short term or rejected them in the long term. Prioritizing non-sexual relationships challenges not only heteronormativity, but what Potts (2002) terms "compulsory sexuality": the notion that we must want to be involved in sexual relationships in some way. As Labuski (2014) argues, however, unlike women who actively embrace an asexual identity, heterosexual women with chronic genital pain often make this "choice" in the context of a heteronormative culture that does not encourage "queering" heterosex, and therefore that simply might close off sexual possibilities.

### Solving Sexual Problems: Medicalized, Biomedicalized, Demedicalized, and Do-It-Yourself Approaches

Given the overall hold of heterosexual norms, it is not surprising that the majority of participants sought some form of sex "expert" advice or therapy for their sexual problems, even if many went on to critique, reject, or deem it ineffective. With or without the label of "female sexual dysfunction" or a one-size-fits-all sexual pharmaceutical drug, middle-class participants in particular were able to access various therapeutic regimes for their perceived sexual problems. A key finding is that medicalized, biomedicalized, demedicalized, and even do-it-yourself options often share key commonalities and depend on one another. Suggesting that the line between these arenas is not as cut and dried as medicalization theory often maintains, medical solutions occasionally involve body work, whereas what often are deemed "alternative" or "complimentary" solutions sometimes involve the purchase of pills. Grassroots self-help groups are used frequently as forums for sharing information about medical therapies.

Medicalization has potential benefits, particularly for women with chronic genital pain – indeed, participants who were told by various doctors that such problems were "all in their head" were particularly grateful for the validation that medicalization provides. Sexual medicine specialists and pelvic physiotherapists alike have developed visual, educational strategies that encourage women to connect to the look, feel, and function of their bodies. Participants enthusiastically described these techniques as increasing their sense of sexual self-awareness and control as they learned that their vagina was an active, rather than a passive, organ.

Although many of these therapies challenge romantic ideologies of "natural" and "essential" sexuality, it is important to keep in mind that therapeutic culture, whether of the "self-help" or face-to-face variety, tends to emphasize individual experience (Becker, 2004). Feminist authors have even critiqued 1970s feminist consciousness-raising sessions as overemphasizing "the self" and individualizing and depoliticizing gender issues (see, for example, Hawkes, 1996). Indeed, within these professionally led consciousness-raising sessions, women's sense of lack of control over sexual encounters were not contextualized in relation to wider gender inequalities – for instance, women's well-documented struggle to articulate their own desires in heterosexual interactions (see Gavey. 1993, 2005; Holland et al. 1994, 1998; Thompson 1990, 1995; Tolman, 2001). Addressing sexual problems one body at a time, even if boosting an individual's sense of empowerment, disguises the socially constructed aspects of culturally defined norms and, arguably, inhibits socio-political, collective action, as seen in participants' unwillingness to share their experiences with their friends. It is also questionable that an expert is necessary to lead these exercises in the first place, and yet they seem to minimize the notion that a woman could desensitize on her own, aside from the assignment of "homework" under professional guidance.

I have also discussed evidence of what Light (2000) refers to as "countervailing powers" that serve as barriers to the (bio)medicalization of sex. Some general practitioners simply did not take women's sexual problems seriously, thereby shutting down that avenue of medicalization, or were so rough with their patients' bodies during examinations that their patients put a stop to the process. The sexual medicine unit at Vancouver's main hospital is one of the few resources dedicated to dealing with sexual complaints that is covered under British Columbia's universal health care plan, but a certain degree of social capital likely is required to access a referral to this resource in the first place. Moreover, once in the system, waiting lists are long and support is not ongoing. Participants considered private sector services such as pelvic physiotherapy simply too expensive. Therefore, many participants had given up on professional advice and forged their own paths when they felt that medical approaches were too inaccessible and costly or deemed them too laborious, traumatic, and/or "unnatural." The scepticism about drugs expressed by this particular group of women is evidence that a sexual pharmaceutical would not easily replace some of the better-liked, low-tech therapies.

## Medicalization and Heteronormativity: A Reciprocal Relationship

In this book I have highlighted the circular and reciprocal relationship between medicalization and heteronormativity. The argument that medical and sexual advice experts tend to validate normative definitions of heterosex is not new. Feminist authors critiquing the field of sexology have long argued that "experts" legitimate and normalize certain modes of sexual expression, and brand all other activities or behaviour as deviant (Gerhard, 2000; Hawkes, 1996; Irvine, 1990; Nicolson, 1993). In this case, the medicalization of "female sexual dysfunction" and the search for a sexual pharmaceutical drug for women is underpinned by key assumptions regarding heterosex. Even Basson's alternative female sexual response cycle (2000d), lauded as taking into consideration individual and interpersonal factors that might inhibit women's spontaneous sexual desire, normalizes an active male sex drive and a passive, but amenable, female sexual response.

In a number of cases, the sex experts I Interviewed supported an intolerant attitude towards women's inability or unwillingness to mirror heterosexual norms. An excellent example is the labelling and treatment of chronic sexual pain, for which the sexual advice practitioners focused their efforts on teaching patients to have penetrative sex using techniques such as vaginal dilators, biofeedback, hypnosis, counselling, and various "homework" activities. The general consensus among these practitioners is that heterosexuality should be worked upon, honed, improved, and mastered through skill building and mental and physical discipline. Indeed, building on Duncombe and Marsden's (1996) theory of relationship-based "sex work," I have demonstrated that women must undertake a "labour of love" to meet exacting heterosexual ideals. Self-help books, women's magazines, and sex manuals also pressure women to work on sexual improvement (as noted by Gupta & Cacchioni, 2013; Jackson & Scott, 1997; Tyler, 2004), but the importance of sex work was also conveyed to the participants in my study rather forcefully during face-to-face visits with doctors and other sexual advice professionals. Sex experts advocate what I have termed "discipline work" as crucial for the longevity of heterosexual relationships; they normalize, but do not celebrate, "performance work"; and they condemn "avoidance work." They frame their advice as being in the best interest of the client, patient, or couple, but career or financial interest also might inform their approach.

Among the more novel of my findings might be the qualitative evidence that the pressure of normative heterosexuality – that is, to perform sexually in a particular manner – helped impel participants in the study to seek "expert" advice, thereby exposing them to "expert" discourses and strategies for treatment in the first place. In part because discourses and structures of heterosexuality made participants feel their status as women depended on their ability to mirror dominant (mainly hetero) sexual norms, they were reluctant to turn to friends as a trusted and valued source of advice or validation. As a result of wider social and economic pressures, women in long-term heterosexual relationships engaged in "sex work," but so did single women and women in short-term relationships. Although  men might also engage in sex work, the women in this study certainly seemed to take on the responsibility of working on heterosex as their duty, sometimes on the advice of their male partners. In a sense, the sex experts were right to warn women that they might be "dumped" for failing to work on their problems with sex, even when their partners did not seem to want to do their share of this work, as in fact many were left by their partners.

The medicalization of women's sexual problems will continue even in the absence of the anticipated "pink" Viagra. Medicalization and the social construction of normative heterosexuality have long been intertwined, and they will continue to sustain each other as long as frequent (hetero) sex ending in orgasm is imbued with the cultural significance it currently enjoys. As examined in historical studies highlighting women's engagement with expert-recommended therapies and self-help, and in existing sociological research exploring women's emotional and sex work, working to achieve heterosexual norms, with or without the direct help of experts, is an established pattern for women that predates pharmaceutical interventions in their sexual enjoyment.

I also considered the argument that challenging heterosexual norms is a way to challenge medicalization. In theorizing the medicalization of sex, the focus typically has been on how the medical community has labelled non-conforming subjects as deviant and has them treated as such. However, the participants in my study who did not seek expert advice for their sexual problems were the most likely to attempt to queer heterosexuality. It is possible that, by avoiding expert sexual advice, they were better able to forge their own path. Obviously, it would be dangerous to assume that we always have the autonomous choice to avoid or embrace the medical paradigm. If medicalization is a form of "social control," as Conrad (1992) and others have argued, it seems that economic and social capital affect the ability both to afford and to reject medicalization. Moreover, it would be naive to believe that medicalization is entirely avoidable in Western urban industrial society, so steeped are lay understandings in this paradigm.

Finally, it remains to be seen if "queering" heterosex or deprioritizing sexual interactions and relationships firmly disrupts the institution of heterosexuality. It is still a matter of debate whether the refusal of the labour of sexual improvement represents a truly subversive act or is just another set of "life politics" (Giddens, 1991) focused on the individual body, rather than structural change or collective emancipation. Particularly for heterosexual-identified women with chronic genital pain who opt out of sexual relationships all together, it is questionable whether many deprioritize sex in the absence of an asexual identity from an agentic place or simply due to a sense of the lack of alternatives (unlike asexual-indentified individuals who actively take on this identity). Either way, women who give up or reject heterosex might face material consequences.

The past few decades of feminist thought have been dominated largely by post-structuralist (Hollway, 1984; McNay, 1992; Weedon, 1987), and "queer" (Butler, 1990, Dollimore, 1991; Fuss, 1991) perspectives, highlighting the interconnections between discourse and power, but also our ability actively to reshape or reinscribe our understandings of gender and sexuality with new meanings and agency. These possibilities have been integral to feminist reimaginings of the "pleasures" of sexualities (Vance, 1984). Indeed, many women are able to realize sexual pleasures with varying levels of agency. However, the case of heterosexual women who do not readily or easily enjoy sex provides one of many cautionary tales about jumping too readily at optimistic possibilities that tend to assume an equal level of structural freedom with men, as well as among and between women. Numerous women in this study from a range of backgrounds had faced sexual, physical, and emotional violence. Many were financially dependent on their male partner, and faced an economic struggle when they were dumped or ended their sexual relationship as a result of their perceived sexual inadequacies. Their strategies for dealing with sexual difficulties thus were deeply embedded in the structures of heterosexuality, patriarchy, colonialism, and capitalism.

If a sexual pharmaceutical drug for women is ever developed and successfully marketed, women will choose whether or not to take the drug in the context of limited options. I therefore must concur with Jackson and Scott (1997), who argued almost twenty years ago that we can "chart shifts" but not "radical ruptures with the past" when it comes to women's material position of equality (p. 552). In addition to changes in sexual patterns and possibilities, greater changes in power relationships associated with gender and other intersecting aspects of identity will be necessary for any radical disruption of "the labour of love."

# Epilogue: The Sexual Pharmaceutical Industry and Its Discontents

Liz Canner's exposé of the sexual pharmaceutical industry, *Orgasm Inc* (2011), includes a warning to viewers regarding its possible side effects, which "may cause uncontrollable laughter, feelings of outrage, followed by symptoms of withdrawal when the film ends." I have experienced all of the above over the past fifteen years of studying, analysing, and speaking out against the politics of what is often so benignly termed the search for a "pink" Viagra. Canner's documentary follows the rise and fall of a potential sex drug for women called Alista, developed by a small Silicon Valley biotech company named Vivus. She was hired to select and edit pornography that clinical trial participants would view while connected to a vaginal plethysmograph that would measure their arousal after having blindly taken either the drug or a placebo.

The story of Alista is telling of the politics of the sexual pharmaceutical industry as a whole. Just before Viagra was released to blockbuster fame, Vivus had a brief heyday of financial success with MUSE (Medicated Urethral System for Erection), a device used to administer a suppository with alprostadil, a vasodilator that increases blood flow to the penis. When Viagra was released just months later as an easy-to-take pill with the same endpoint, Vivus stock dropped dramatically. As chronicled in Canner's film, Vivus wasted no time in attempting to piggyback the success of its alprostadil medication onto women, and testing began soon after on Alista. Despite the endless massaging of endpoints as captured on film, the company simply was unable to demonstrate that Alista had any meaningful benefit greater than the placebo. To add insult to injury, Canner had candidly captured on film the lengths the company had gone to, bringing to life the ethical problems associated with a public company's taking responsibility for our sexual pleasure and safety from drug side effects.

Now, years later, alprostadil, the main ingredient of Alista, is rising from the ashes thanks to a San Diego biotech company named Apricus Biosciences, which has promised better delivery of this vasodilator using a skin-penetration enhancer called dodecyl 2(N,N-dimethylamino)-propionate. Presto: we now have Vitaros for men and Femprox for women, currently under clinical trials with the hope of being launched in Canada, the United States, and Europe by Abbott Laboratories. When researching information about these drugs, I was struck by Apricus's blatantly commercial tone. The very first line of a "corporate strategy" document, published online, boldly "announces its corporate goals for 2013," which include focusing its *"corporate strategy on its high value assets such as Vitaros for erectile dysfunction ('ED') and Femprox for female sexual arousal disorder ('FSAD')."* And a few sentences later, "The Board of Directors believes that the *greatest potential for shareholder value creation is in the further development and commercialization, through strategic partnerships, of the Company's primary commercial and pipeline assets, particularly Vitaros* (alprostadil 0.3% topical cream) *and Femprox* (alprostadil 0.4% topical cream) *for male and female sexual health"* (Apricus Biosciences, 2013, para. 1; emphasis added).

However, the sexual pharmaceutical industry and the wider medicalization of sexuality continue to provoke critical response. The New View has grown over time, tackling more areas of sexual medicalization. The main focus of the campaign over the past five years has been social forces and the manipulative marketing tactics fuelling the growing trend of female genital cosmetic surgery such as labiaplasty and vaginal "tightening" and "rejuvenation" surgeries. In 2008 New View members organized a street protest outside the offices of a New York City cosmetic genital surgeon; in 2009 an arts and crafts political event titled "Vulvagraphics" was held in celebration of genital diversity; in 2010 a "counter-conference" was organized to the second annual meeting of cosmetic genital surgeons in Las Vegas, Nevada; and in 2011 came the launch of the "Vulvanomics" campaign. This campaign included a petition protesting the marketing techniques used by many surgeons; the petition was later sent to the US Federal Trade Commission's Office of Consumer Affairs and the American College of Obstetrics and Gynecology. Vulvanomics also included a letter-writing campaign whereby people wrote directly to surgeons to protest their "before" and "after" images (see Braun 2009, 2010).

In 2011, inspired by the Flibanserin hearing, I organized an international, interdisciplinary conference on wider trends in the Medicalization of Sex, with Leonore Tiefer as one of the keynote speakers.[1] Approximately two hundred people from all over Canada, the United States, South America, Europe, Australia, New Zealand, and Israel gathered in Vancouver to question science, medicine, and the pharmaceutical industry's efforts to shape our understandings and experiences of sexuality. Included in this group were cross-generational, junior, and senior scholars from all branches of the humanities and social sciences, doctors, nurses, counsellors, therapists, women's health advocates, sex educators, journalists, and creative artists. Speaking on a plethora of topics, presenters questioned medical conceptions of sexual "normality" and "deviancy," "function" and "dysfunction," "hygiene" and "pollution," and "risk" and "safety." There was much concern regarding the use of precious resources to measure sexuality – through population studies, surveys, questionnaires, scales, rulers, clinical diagnosis, plethysmographs, and functional magnetic resonance imaging – at a time when quality sex education continues to be difficult to access and evidence supports the need for deepening, rather than shrinking, definitions of sexual "normality." The presentations demonstrated once again that the rationalization and quantification of sexuality is by no means an objective process, but one that is often driven by profit and career expansion. Papers on trans* issues provided a welcome critical intervention as theorists discussed the dual role medical technologies play in trans* lives, both funnelling diverse identities into narrow medical models and offering transformative possibilities through pharmaceuticals and surgeries (see, for example, Elliot, 2010). Later, Tiefer and I co-edited a special issue of the *Journal of Sex Research* on "The Medicalization of Sex," with the intention of tackling new audiences, rather than simply "preaching to the choir" (Cacchioni & Tiefer, 2011; 2012).

Tiefer and I reconvened at the 2013 Selling Sickness: People Before Profits conference she convened in Washington, DC, along with Kim Witczak, a woman who became interested in medicalization when her husband committed suicide as a result of an undisclosed drug side effect. As described in the *British Medical Journal*, this was a "self funded grassroots conference [that] deliberately sought to model the possibility of a new social health movement with equal representation of professional and advocate perspectives and extended time for discussion" (Tiefer, Witczak, & Heath, 2013. p. 1). A "Call to Action on Selling Sickness," drafted and endorsed by attendees and others after the conference, expresses concern over "the problems of biased science, hidden data, inflated diagnostic categories, unnecessary screening and treatment, and the widespread neglect of social factors when treating illness." It aims to put "an end to direct-to-consumer advertising of diagnostics and drugs, ensure appropriate testing of new drugs and devices, put forward reform of the patent system, and promote responsible health journalism."[2]

The New View is now challenging the "Even the Score Campaign," a petition circulated by a group of "consumer advocates," four congresswomen, and various drug companies (including Sprout) demanding that the US Food and Drug Administration (FDA) approve a sexual pharmaceutical for women.[3] "Even the Score" is a plea for equality based on the claim that twenty-six sex drugs have been approved for men's sexual dysfunction. This statistic, which has been taken up as legitimate in most popular media coverage, is an exaggerated number, counting singular drugs in various dosages or formulations as more than one drug and including reference to drugs that are used *off-label* for the treatment of men's sexual problems. The campaign, in fact, flaunts the logic of neoliberal, "choice feminism," which portrays gender inequalities as individual issues, solvable by access to more consumer choices. In this case, equality is framed as equal access to an equal number of drug choices, without any scrutiny over the safety or efficacy of these drugs. The New View petition against "Even the Score" urges, "Don't be fooled by PR flim-flam dressed up in the language of women's rights. Let's support the FDA and demand that Big Pharma cancel its fraudulent PR campaigns."

Although the critique of the medicalization of sex is ongoing and remains significant, there are numerous gaps in research activism in this area. When I teach about sexual medicalization at the University of Victoria, my students and I continually return to these questions: Who is targeted in the pharmaceutical research agenda? who is explicitly disregarded? in which ways? and to what end? how do race, class, sexuality, ability, gender conformity, and non-conformity feature into this discussion? What can queer, trans*, cyborg, and post-human theorizations of the body tell us about our embodiment, medicalized or not? And what can feminist critics of sexual medicalization learn from disability theorists and activists, who have long contended with the limits of heteronormative constructions of sex?

As a sign of defensiveness in the midst of all of this critical engagement, but also as part of their ongoing quest for legitimacy, the physicians who make up the  International Society for the Study of Women's Sexual Health, a heavily Pharma-funded group, have sparked a campaign called "Your Voice, Your WISH" (Women's Initiative for Sexual Health). The WISH campaign, as it is known, is an emotionally fuelled and misleading convergence of Big Pharma propaganda, disease mongering, and faux-feminist rhetoric. Shamelessly, the campaign perpetuates the fact that "43% of women suffer from some form of sexual dysfunction," despite the critique of this statistic in numerous articles and books, including by the author of the original study on which the statistic is based (Moynihan & Mintzes, 2010). Paralleling "pinkwashing" breast cancer propaganda (King, 2006), the campaign website[4] features a video montage of male and female doctors. Phrases such as "sex is the spice of life," "WISH for equality," and "TRUST WOMEN" are scrawled across forearms and hands while saccharine music plays in the background. The video ends with the sentiment, "sign your support today," signalling a petition to endorse three wishes:

- My WISH is that my sexual health be viewed as an integral part of my overall health and well being, not a "lifestyle" choice.
- My WISH is that women who suffer from sexual dysfunction be respectfully evaluated for the best course of treatment, whether medical or psychological, not dismissed.
- My WISH is that, provided a therapy is safe and effective, government agencies strongly consider approval of a treatment option for women just as they have for men.

These wishes are emblematic of the times: sexual "function" has been constructed as a matter of "health" and "dysfunction" a matter of illness. Doctors are drawing on tactics used in embodied health campaigns and LGBTQ rights activism to argue that having female sexual dysfunction or hypoactive sexual desire disorder is not a "lifestyle choice" but a biological fact.

And yet, without skipping a beat, Leonore Tiefer was quick to condemn this campaign on the Selling Sickness website: "Your Voice, Your Wish claims to know what women want, sexually, and – guess what, what they want is not better sex education, not safer contraception, not better sex partners, not less sexual violence, not less sexual objectification – not even affordable childcare so they wouldn't be so tired – but more medicine … If women of the world were given 3 wishes for a better sex life, who besides brazen agents of selling sickness would say they'd choose treatments and therapies?" Thinking of all the women I interviewed about their experience of treatments and therapies, I have to agree. Although many engaged in the labour of love as an immediate way of dealing with sexual dissatisfactions, their wishes were much deeper.

# Appendix: Participants' Profiles

(Profiles are in alphabetical order, followed by age/race/ethnicity/ nationality/occupation/religion/sexuality/relationship status *as self-described by the participants* in a qualitative questionnaire, with pseudonyms chosen to ensure anonymity.)

**Amy**, 29, white, Canadian, physiotherapist, heterosexual, long-term partner.

**Anna**, 34, Dutch, South African, actress/writer, heterosexual, born-again Christian, married.

**Celia**, 56, Chinese, Canadian, nurse, heterosexual, divorced, single, two grown children.

**Charlene**, 27, white, Canadian, airport ground staff employee, heterosexual, lives with long-term partner.

**Courtney**, 25, white, Canadian, university programs and promotions officer, heterosexual, lives with long-term sexual partner.

**Danielle**, 44, white, Canadian, dental hygienist instructor, heterosexual, married.

**Elizabeth**, 57, white, Canadian, art student/retired counsellor, heterosexual, married, full-time care of one child.

**Faye**, 42, white, New Zealander, assistant store manager, heterosexual, divorced, now single, part-time care of three children.

**Grace**, 53, Chinese, Canadian, cruise consultant, heterosexual, divorced twice, once widowed, single.

**Hannah**, 53, German, Canadian, formerly owned a small business, now a university student, heterosexual, divorced, single, full-time care of two children.

**Jas**, 27, Indian, Punjabi, Canadian, yoga instructor/video store employee, heterosexual, single.

**Jolene**, 51, Indigenous, Musqueam, Canadian, gas station attendant, heterosexual, single, two grown children.

**Julie**, 27, white, Canadian, office manager, bisexual, lives with long-term male partner.

**Kate**, 43, white, Canadian, heterosexual, married, full-time care of two children.

**Simone**, 30, Eurasian, Canadian, escort, bisexual, lives with long-term male partner, full-time care of one child.

**Lauren**, 21, white, Canadian, heterosexual, university student, in first sexual relationship with long-term partner.

**Leanne**, 29, white, Canadian, environmental science researcher, lesbian, divorced former male partner, recently married to female partner.

**Linda**, 26, white, Canadian, lab technician/personal trainer, about to begin medical school, heterosexual, lives with long-term partner.

**Lindsay**, 39, white, Canadian, nurse, heterosexual, single.

**Louise**, 35, white, Canadian, office manager, heterosexual, remarried, full-time care of two children from first marriage.

**Lucy**, 29, white, Canadian, French school teacher, heterosexual, long-term partner.

**Maria**, 22, Italian, Canadian, university student/waitress, heterosexual, single.

**Mika**, 27, Japanese, Canadian, cashier at a book store, heterosexual, single.

**Monica**, 47, Chinese, Canadian, part-time holistic aesthetician, heterosexual, divorced, single, full-time care of two young children.

**Nicola**, 34, white, Canadian, former janitor, recently became school teacher, heterosexual, divorced, now in long-term relationship.

**Olivia**, 37, Latina, Mexican Canadian, Catholic, owner of communication design company, heterosexual, married.

**Samantha**, 24, white, American, actress/ESL teacher, heterosexual, lives with long-term partner.

**Sarah**, 25, white, Canadian, broadcast journalism student, heterosexual, lives with long-term partner.

**Sophie**, 32, white, British, part-time arts administrator, heterosexual, single.

**Susan**, 62, Japanese, Canadian, retired lab technician, heterosexual, married, two grown children.

**Zoe**, 34, white, Canadian, radio documentary maker, bisexual, lives with long-term male partner, trying to get pregnant.

# Notes

**Preface**

1 Phase-3 clinical trials are intended as the final tests of a drug's safety and efficacy prior to its submission to regulatory authorities for approval.
2 According to the Draft Guidance for Industry Female Sexual Dysfunction: Clinical Development of Drug Products for Treatment (United States, 2000),

> primary endpoints for trials of drug products to treat FSD ... should be based on the number of successful and satisfactory sexual events or encounters over time. The determination of *successful* and *satisfactory* should be made by the woman participating in the trial, as opposed to her partner. Such *events* or *encounters* include:
> satisfactory sexual intercourse;
> sexual intercourse resulting in orgasm;
> oral sex resulting in orgasm; and
> partner-initiated or self masturbation resulting in orgasm.

> Thus, while claiming to authorize women to self-define what an SSE might entail, the definition assumes it will involve intercourse and/or orgasm.

**Introduction**

1 Seminal texts on these theories reference works by Tiefer and other critics of the politics of the sexual pharmaceutical era as providing a classic case study in biomedicalization. In turn, critics such as Tiefer (2012) and Marshall (2012), writing on the politics of the sexual pharmaceutical industry, increasingly use the concept of "biomedicalization" to explain the growing

power of drug companies to define and shape medical and popular understandings of health and illness.

2 According to Hollway (1984), the *male sex drive* refers to the discursive construction of men as biologically motivated by a strong urge towards the coital and orgasmic imperative. By contrast, women's sexuality has been theorized traditionally in binary opposition to men's sexuality through the *have/hold* discourse, a term Hollway intentionally worded to evoke its connection to Christian family values. This discourse constructs women as valuing sex as a means to emotional connection and reproduction, rather than physical pleasure. The *permissive* discourse is theoretically gender neutral, a product of the insistence that all humans are sexual beings, as popularized during the period known as the "sexual revolution."

3 Evans, Riley, and Shankar (2010) also examine "technologies of sexiness" and the wider work on the formation of the sexualized subject.

## 1. The Rise and Decline of Big Pharma's "Sexual Revolution"

1 There are subtle differences in these drugs in relation to how long and how quickly they work.

2 See "Is It [LowT]?" available online at http://www.isitlowt.com/.

3 As profiled in Liz Canner's film *Orgasm Inc.* (2011), another sexual pharmaceutical hopeful for women involving the vascular system was Alista. After much hype, however, clinical trials did not produce a meaningful benefit. As discussed in the Epilogue, Femprox, a compound that uses the same main ingredient as Alista but a different delivery method, is now in being tested as a treatment for FSAD.

4 See the Eros Therapy Web site, http://www.eros-therapy.com/index. cfm?optionid=522#freemovie, accessed 29 January 2013.

5 "LibiGel, Viagra for Women or Just Another Testosterone Cream?" Available online at http://www.libigel.org/.

6 This was not the first brain drug for an FSD subset to be conceived. There have been high hopes for a nasal spray of bremelanotide, branded as PT-141. Scientists argue that this spray enhances sexual functioning in men and women by going "to the brain itself" (Dibbell, 2006, para. 5), but the FDA has not yet approved the drug. In fact, the maker, Palatin Inc., delayed a late-state study because the FDA had serious concerns about the research design of the drug trial. In phase-two-B trials, bremelanotide showed an increase in the number of sexually satisfying events by 0.8 (2.9) with a 1.75 mg dose and by 0.7 (2.4) with a 1.25 mg dose versus the

placebo (2.3), a measure determined subjectively by each participant. These results are minimal, but the placebo effect is impressive. Side effects in this case included mild-to-moderate facial flushing, nausea, emesis, and increased blood pressure.

7  See http://trimelpharmaceuticals.com/.

8  Even with a dip in sales of Viagra and issues with Pfizer's patent, Pfizer continues to dream up new ways of profiting from this compound. Sildenafil citrate is now used off-label on men and women undergoing fertility treatments. A Pfizer-funded pilot study of twenty-five men (Jannini, Lombardo, Salacone, Gandini, & Lenzi, 2004) came to the obvious conclusion that men with erectile difficulties were more likely to be able to obtain and sustain an erection for the purpose of giving a sperm sample. A questionnaire audit of the Human Fertilization and Embryo Authority's licensed conception units in the United Kingdom showed that 42 per cent would prescribe sildenafil to patients with difficulty producing semen samples on demand (Glenn, McVicar, McClure, & Lewis, 2007). However, Glenn et al. (2007) have conducted extensive research to suggest that the use of sildenafil impairs pre-implantation and post-implantation embryo development. Met with a great deal of media hype, research has also been conducted on the effect of intra-vaginal use of sildenafil to improve uterine artery blood flow and to thicken the endometrial lining during in-vitro fertilization treatment (Paulus, Strehler, Zhang, Jelinkova, El-Danasouri, & Sterzik, 2002; Sher & Fisch, 2000). Paulus et al. (2002) admit, however, that the "correlation between pregnancy rate and endometrial thickness or uterine artery blood flow remains controversial" (p. 847).

9  See http://newshe.com/.

10  The seeds of Tiefer's anti-medicalization activism were sown by the 1992 National Institutes of Health Consensus Development Conference on "Impotence," which she describes as a "watershed event in the progress of the medicalization of sexuality and the dismantling of the psycho-bio-social approach" (Tiefer, 2007, p. 475). Aware that the aim of the conference was to validate impotence as a primarily physiological issue with some psychological "risk factors" (p. 476), despite much sexological research to suggest otherwise, she suggested that the report be published in the *International Journal of Impotence Research* alongside commentary from sexologists and urologists. She even provided the names of thirty-one sexologists she hoped would "weigh in with trenchant commentaries about the dangers of the rush towards medicalization." Unfortunately, her colleagues disappointed – only fourteen responded, none with any fervent critique.

## 2. Treating Women's Sexual Pain

1 To this day, women who experience this type of pain deem months and even years of being misdiagnosed or not diagnosed at all as one the most distressing aspects of the pain itself (Feldhaus-Dahir, 2011).
2 Recently, the DSM-5 has revised these definitions to reflect a single diagnostic category of sexual pain disorders called "genito-pelvic pain/penetration disorder."
3 See Peter Pacik's website at http://www.plasticsurgerypa.com/about-peter-t-pacik-md-facs/.
4 See http://www.vaginismusmd.com/about/peter-bio/.
5 See http://www.neogyn.us/neogyn-cutaneous-lysate; accessed 12 February 2012.
6 In Cacchioni and Wolkowitz (2011), we examine how sexual medicine specialists and pelvic physiotherapists negotiated the paradox of touching women's painful genitals in an effort to lead them to pleasure.
7 Currently there seems to be no published research examining the experiences of women who have participated in desensitization therapy with a male practitioner. Likewise, I know of no research examining the perspectives of male therapists in this field.
8 See http://www.comeasyouare.com/default/index.cfm/sex-tips/sex-how-tos/silicone-dilators-and-dilation-exercises.
9 See http://www.healpelvicpain.com.
10 See http://www.beyondbasicsphysicaltherapy.com/pfd.
11 See http://vaginismus-awareness-network.org/. Unfortunately the site is no longer online, but the material formerly posted is nonetheless worthy of discussion.

## 3. The Limits of Normative Heterosex

1 It is important to note that the comments on "porn" made by participants in this study referred directly to heterosexual, mainstream pornography, and reflected only their sentiments on the negative consequences of viewing porn. Numerous feminist authors have written about the political importance of feminist heterosexual and LGBTQ porn and the possible pleasures of mainstream porn (see Busby, 2004; Kipnis, 2006).
2 Recently, Mount Holyoke College in Massachusetts cancelled a production of *The Vagina Monologues* for not being trans* inclusive (Voss, 2015). Eve Ensler, author and director of the play, issued the following statement: "*The Vagina Monologues* never intended to be a play about what it means to

be a woman. It is and always has been a play about what it means to have a vagina. In the play, I never defined a woman as a person with a vagina" (para. 4).

3 Julie, self-defined as bisexual, did not comment on sexual experiences with women.

## 5. Refusing Heteronormative Sex Work

1 Although Butler (1990) believes that "identity categories tend to be instruments of regulatory regimes," (p. 13), she allows that "queer" can be a "discursive rallying point" for various sexual groups, including "bisexuals and straights for whom the term expresses an affiliation with an anti-homophobic politics" (Butler, 1993, p. 547).

2 See http://www.asexuality.org/home/; accessed 18 December 2012.

3 "Lesbian bed death" is a term used to describe low levels of sexual activity in long-term lesbian relationships. It was first used in lay vernacular in the 1980s, but was later taken up by sex therapists and sex researchers (see, for example, Hall, 2001; Iasenza, 2001). Many understand the term to imply that lesbians are particularly susceptible to a waning sex life as a result of their gender. However, the normalization of this term (and phenomenon) also might give lesbian couples licence to embrace an ebbing and flowing sex life in ways that are expected to be alarming by heteronormative standards.

## Epilogue

1 Other experts on the medicalization of sex who also gave talks include keynote speaker Jennifer Terry and plenary speakers Virginia Braun, Liz Canner, Carol Groneman, Barbara Marshall, Elizabeth Reis, Judy Segal, and Rebecca Jordan Young.

2 See http://sellingsickness.com/final-statement/.

3 See http://eventhescore.org/.

4 See https://www.yourvoiceyourwish.com/.

# References

Angel, K. (2012). Contested psychiatric ontology and feminist critique: "Female sexual dysfunction" and the diagnostic and statistical manual. *History of the Human Sciences, 25*(4), 3–24. http://dx.doi.org/10.1177/09526 95112456949

Angelmar, R., Angelmar, S., & Kane, L. (2007). Building strong condition brands. *Journal of Medical Marketing, 7*(4), 341–351. http://dx.doi.org/10.1057/palgrave.jmm.5050101

American Psychiatric Association. (2000). *Diagnostic and statistical manual of mental disorders* (Revised 4th ed.). Washington, DC: American Psychiatric Association.

American Psychiatric Association. (2013). *Diagnostic and statistical manual of mental disorders* (5th ed.). Washington, DC: American Psychiatric Association.

Apricus Biosciences. (2013, January 3). Apricus Biosciences announces corporate goals for 2013. Retrieved from http://ir.apricusbio.com/phoenix.zhtml?c=118007&p=irol-newsArticle&ID=1981204

Ayling, K., & Ussher, J. M. (2008). "If sex hurts, am I still a woman?" The subjective experience of vulvodynia in hetero-sexual women. *Archives of Sexual Behavior, 37*(2), 294–304. http://dx.doi.org/10.1007/s10508-007-9204-1

Basson, R. (2001a). Are the complexities of women's sexual function reflected in the new consensus definitions of dysfunction? *Journal of Sex & Marital Therapy, 27*(2), 105–112. http://dx.doi.org/10.1080/00926230152051725

Basson, R. (2001b). Human sex-response cycles. *Journal of Sex & Marital Therapy, 27*(1), 33–43. http://dx.doi.org/10.1080/00926230152035831

Basson, R. (2001c). Using a different model for female sexual response to address women's problematic low sexual desire. *Journal of Sex & Marital Therapy, 27*(5), 395–403. http://dx.doi.org/10.1080/713846827

Basson, R. (2002a). Are our definitions of women's desire, arousal, and sexual pain disorders too broad and our definition of orgasmic disorder too narrow? *Journal of Sex & Marital Therapy, 28*(4), 289–300. http://dx.doi.org/10.1080/00926230290001411

Basson, R. (2002b). The complexities of female sexual arousal disorder: Potential role of pharmacotherapy. *World Journal of Urology, 20*(2), 119–126. http://dx.doi.org/10.1007/s00345-002-0273-4

Basson, R. (2002c). Rethinking low sexual desire in women. *BJOG: An International Journal of Obstetrics and Gynecology, 109*(4), 357–363. http://dx.doi.org/10.1111/j.1471-0528.2002.01002.x

Basson, R. (2002d). Women's sexual desire: Disordered or misunderstood? *Journal of Sex & Marital Therapy, 28*(1), 17–28. http://dx.doi.org/10.1080/00926230252851168

Basson, R. (2005). Women's sexual dysfunction: Revised and expanded definitions. *Canadian Medical Association Journal, 172*(10), 1327–1333. http://dx.doi.org/10.1503/cmaj.1020174

Basson, R. (2008). Women's sexual function and dysfunction: Current uncertainties, future directions. *International Journal of Impotence Research, 20*(5), 466–478. http://dx.doi.org/10.1038/ijir.2008.23

Basson, R., Berman, J., Burnett, A., Derogatis, L., Ferguson, D., et al. (2001). Report of the international consensus development conference on female sexual dysfunction: Definitions and classifications. *Journal of Sex & Marital Therapy, 27*(2), 83–94. http://dx.doi.org/10.1080/00926230152051707

Basson, R., McInnes, R., Smith, M. D., Hodgson, G., & Koppiker, N. (2002). Efficacy and safety of sildenafil citrate in women with sexual dysfunction associated with female sexual arousal disorder. *Journal of Women's Health & Gender-Based Medicine, 11*(4), 367–377. http://dx.doi.org/10.1089/152460902317586001

Basson, R., Wierman, M. E., van Lankveld, J., & Brotto, L. (2010). Summary of the recommendations on sexual dysfunctions in women. *Sexual Medicine, 7*(1pt2), 314–326. http://dx.doi.org/10.1111/j.1743-6109.2009.01617.x

Beasley, C., Brook, H., & Holmes, M. (2012). *Heterosexuality in theory and practice*. New York, NY: Routledge.

Becker, S (2004). The myth of empowerment: Women and the therapeutic culture in America. New York, NY: New York University Press.

Berens, J. (2001, May 6). Sisters are doing it for themselves. *Guardian*. Retrieved from http://www.theguardian.com/theobserver/2001/may/06/life1.lifemagazine1

Berman, J., Berman, L., & Bumiller, E. (2001). *For women only: A revolutionary guide to overcoming sexual dysfunction and reclaiming your sex life*. New York, NY: Henry Holt.

Berman, L. (2004, September 27). Not in the mood? Now there's a patch. *Chicago Sun-Times*, pp. 2–6.

Berman, L. (2006). *The passion prescription: Ten weeks to your best sex – ever!* New York: NY Hyperion.

Berman, L. (2008). *Real sex for real women: Intimacy, pleasure, and sexual wellbeing*. London, UK: Dorling Kindersley.

Berman, L. (2009). *The sex bible: Your bedside guide to a lifetime of sexual satisfaction*. London, UK: Dorling Kindersley.

Berman, L. (Interviewer) (2010a). [Radio interview on Oprah Radio with Dr Michael Krychman]. *Women's sex drives*. Retrieved from http://www.oprah.com/oprahradio/Womens-Sex-Drives-Audio

Berman, L. (2010b). *It's not him, it's you! How to take charge of your life and create the love and intimacy you deserve*. London, UK: Dorling Kindersley.

Berman, L. (2010c). *The book of love: Every couple's guide to emotional and sexual intimacy*. London, UK: Dorling Kindersley.

Berman, L. (2011). *Loving Sex*. London, UK: Dorling Kindersley.

Berman, L., Berman, J., & Schweiger, A.B. (2006). *Secrets of the sexually satisfied woman: Ten keys to unlocking ultimate sexual pleasure*. New York, NY: Hyperion.

Binik, Y. (2005). Should dyspareunia be retained as a sexual dysfunction in DSM-V? A painful classification decision. *Archives of Sexual Behavior, 34*(1), 11–21. http://dx.doi.org/10.1007/s10508-005-0998-4

Blakeley, K. (2009). Self-help books: Why women can't stop reading them.... *Forbes.com*. Retrieved from http://www.forbes.com/2009/06/10/self-help-books-relationships-forbes-woman-time-marriage.html

Block, J. (2013, April 30). Will this pill fix your sex life? *Daily Beast*. Retrieved from http://www.thedailybeast.com/newsweek/2013/04/29/will-this-pill-fix-your-sex-life.html

Bogaert, A. (2004). Asexuality: Prevalence and associated factors in a national probability sample. *Journal of Sex Research, 41*(3), 279–287. http://dx.doi.org/10.1080/00224490409552235

Bourdieu, S (19S84). Distinction: A social critique of the judgement of taste. Boston, MA: Harvard University Press.

Both, S., & Everaerd, W. (2002). Comments on "The female sexual response: A different model". *Journal of Sex & Marital Therapy, 28*(1), 11–15. http://dx.doi.org/10.1080/009262302317250972

Boyer, S. C., Goldfinger, C., Thibault-Gagnon, S., & Pukall, C. F. (2011). Management of female sexual pain disorders. In R. Balon (Ed.), *Sexual Dysfunction: Beyond the brain-body connection* (pp. 83–104). New York, NY: Karger.

Bradford, A., & Meston, C. (2009). Placebo response in the treatment of women's sexual dysfunctions: A review and commentary. *Journal of Sex & Marital Therapy, 35*(3), 164–181. http://dx.doi.org/10.1080/00926230802716302

Braithwaite, A. (2002). The personal, the political, third-wave, and post-feminisms. *Feminist Theory*, *3*(3), 335–344. http://dx.doi.org/10.1177/146470002762492033

Bransen, E. (1992). Has menstruation been medicalised? Or will it never happen? *Sociology of Health & Illness*, *14*(1), 98–110. http://dx.doi.org/10.1111/1467-9566.ep11007176

Braun, V. (2009). The women are doing it for themselves: The rhetoric of choice and agency around female genital 'cosmetic' surgery. *Australian Feminist Studies*, *24*(60), 233–249. http://dx.doi.org/10.1080/08164640902852449

Braun, V. (2010). Female genital cosmetic surgery: A critical review of current knowledge and contemporary debates. *Journal of Women's Health*, *19*(7), 1393–1407. http://dx.doi.org/10.1089/jwh.2009.1728

Braun, V., Gavey, N., & McPhillips, K. (2003). The "fair deal"? Unpacking accounts of reciprocity in heterosex. *Sexualities*, *6*(2), 237–261. http://dx.doi.org/10.1177/1363460703006002005

Brennan, S. (2011). Violent victimization of Aboriginal women in the Canadian provinces, 2009. *Juristat: Canadian Centre for Justice Statistics*. Ottawa: Statistics Canada. May. Available online at http://www.statcan.gc.ca/pub/85-002-x/2011001/article/11439-eng.htm.

Brotto, L.A. (2011). Non-judgmental, present-moment, sex … as if your life depended on it. *Sexual and Relationship Therapy*, *26*(3), 215–216. http://dx.doi.org/10.1080/14681994.2011.595402

Brotto, L. A., Knudson, G., Inskip, J., Rhodes, K., & Erskine, Y. (2010). Asexuality: A mixed methods approach. *Archives of Sexual Behavior*, *39*(3), 599–618. http://dx.doi.org/10.1007/s10508-008-9434-x

Brotto, L., & Yule, M. A. (2011). Physiological and subjective sexual arousal in self-identified asexual women. *Archives of Sexual Behavior*, *40*(4), 699–712. http://dx.doi.org/10.1007/s10508-010-9671-7

Brown, H. Gurley (1962). *Sex and the single girl*. New York, NY: Geis.

Bullough, V.L. (1973). Marriage in the Middle Ages, 5: Medieval medical and scientific views of women. *Viator*, *4*(4), 485–501.

Burgess, A. (2005). Queering heterosexual spaces: Positive space campaigns disrupting campus heteronormativity. *Canadian Women's Studies*, *24*, 27–30.

Burrill, K. G. (2009). Queering bisexuality. *Journal of Bisexuality*, *9*(3-4), 491–499. http://dx.doi.org/10.1080/15299710903316737

Busby, K. (2004). The queer sensitive interveners in the Little Sisters case: A response to Dr. Kendall. *Journal of Homosexuality*, *47*(3-4), 129–150. http://dx.doi.org/10.1300/J082v47n03_07

Butler, J. (1990). *Gender trouble: Feminism and the subversion of identity*. New York: Routledge.

Butler, J. (1993). *Bodies that matter*. New York, NY: Routledge.

Cacchioni, T. (2007). Heterosexuality and "the labour of love": A contribution to recent debates of female sexual dysfunction. *Sexualities, 10*(3), 299–320. http://dx.doi.org/10.1177/1363460707078320

Cacchioni, T. (2010). Flibanserin testimony. FDA advisory hearing on Flibanserin. Gaithersburg, MD, June 18.

Cacchioni, T. & Tiefer, L. (2011). Final report on the medicalization of sex conference., Vancouver, BC, 28–30 April.

Cacchioni, T., & Tiefer, L. (2012). Why medicalization? Introduction to the special issue on the medicalization of sex. *Journal of Sex Research, 49*(4), 307–310. http://dx.doi.org/10.1080/00224499.2012.690112

Cacchioni, T., & Wolkowitz, C. (2011). Treating women's sexual difficulties: The bodywork of sexual therapy. *Sociology of Health & Illness, 33*(2), 266–279. http://dx.doi.org/10.1111/j.1467-9566.2010.01288.x

Canner, E. (Director). (2011). *Orgasm Inc* [Documentary]. United States: First Run Features.

Carpenter, L.M. (2002). Gender and the meaning of virginity loss in the contemporary United States. *Gender & Society, 16*, 345–365. http://dx.doi.org/10.1177/0891243202016003005

Carvalho, J., & Nobre, P. (2010). Sexual desire in women: an integrative approach regarding psychological, medical, and relationship dimensions. *Journal of Sexual Medicine, 7*(5), 1807–1815. http://dx.doi.org/10.1111/j.1743-6109.2010.01716.x

Chia, M., Chia, M., Abrams, D., & Abrams, R. C. (2002). *The multi-orgasmic couple: Sexual secrets every couple should know*. New York, NY: HarperOne.

Clarke, A. E., Mamo, L., Fishman, J. R. Shim, J. K., & Fosket, J. R. (2003). Biomedicalization: Technoscientific transformations of health, illness, and US biomedicine. *American Sociological Review, 68*(2), 161–194. http://dx.doi.org/10.2307/1519765

Cobb, J. C. (1997). Outercourse as a safe and sensible alternative to contraceptives. *American Journal of Public Health, 87*(8), 1380–1381. http://dx.doi.org/10.2105/AJPH.87.8.1380

Comfort, A., & Quilliam, S. (2009). *The joy of sex: The timeless guide to lovemaking, ultimate revised edition*. London, UK: Crown.

Conrad, P. (1992). Medicalization and social control. *Annual Review of Sociology, 18*(1), 209–232. http://dx.doi.org/10.1146/annurev.so.18.080192.001233

Conrad, P. (2007). *The medicalization of society: On the transformation of human conditions into treatable disorders*. Baltimore, MD: Johns Hopkins University Press.

Conrad, P., & Leiter, V. (2004). Medicalization, markets and consumers. *Journal of Health and Social Behavior, 45*, 158–176.

Crawford, R. (1980). Healthism and the medicalization of everyday life. *International Journal of Health Services, 10*(3), 365–388. http://dx.doi.org/10.2190/3H2H-3XJN-3KAY-G9NY

Crenshaw, K. (1989). Demarginalizing the intersection of race and sex: A black feminist critique of antidiscrimination doctrine, feminist theory and antiracist politics. *University of Chicago Legal Forum, 140,* 139–168.

Cruikshank, B. (1999). *The will to empower: democratic citizens and other subjects.* Ithaca, NY: Cornell University Press.

Darcé, K. (2007, August 4). A step closer to his dream: Sexual-medicine expert moves to San Diego to get his craft recognized. *San Diego Union-Tribune.* Retrieved from http://www.utsandiego.com/uniontrib/20070804/news_1b4goldstein.html

Davis, K. (2007). Reclaiming women's bodies: Colonialist trope or critical epistemology? *Sociological Review, 55,* 50–64. http://dx.doi.org/10.1111/j.1467-954X.2007.00692.x

Davis, M. (1963). *Sexual responsibility in marriage.* New York: Dial Press.

Davis, M. W. (2003). *The Sex-starved marriage: Boosting your marriage libido: A couple's guide.* New York, NY: Simon & Schuster.

DeLamater, J. D., & Sill, M. (2005). Sexual desire in later life. *Journal of Sex Research, 42*(2), 138–149. http://dx.doi.org/10.1080/00224490509552267

D'Emilio, J., & Freedman, E. B. (1988). *Intimate matters: A history of sexuality in America.* New York, NY: Harper & Row.

Dennerstein, L., Hayes, R., Sand, M., & Lehert, P. (2009). Attitudes toward and frequency of partner interactions among women reporting decreased sexual desire. *Journal of Sexual Medicine, 6*(6), 1668–1673. http://dx.doi.org/10.1111/j.1743-6109.2009.01274.x

Deutsch, H. (1944). *The psychology of women.* New York: Grune & Stratton.

Dibbell, J. (2006, April 23). Let us spray. *Observer.* Retrieved from http://www.theguardian.com/science/2006/apr/23/medicineandhealth.observermagazine

Digby, A. (1989). Women's biological straightjacket. In J. Mendus & J. Rendall (Eds.), *Sexuality and subordination: Interdisciplinary studies of gender in the nineteenth century* (pp. 192–220). London, UK: Routledge.

Dollimore, J. (1991). *Sexual dissidence.* Oxford, UK: Oxford University Press. http://dx.doi.org/10.1093/acprof:oso/9780198112259.001.0001

Dubowitz, N., Puretz, M., & Fugh-Berman, A. (2012, August 20). Low-T, high profit? [Web log post.] *Bioethics Forum.* Message posted to http://www.thehastingscenter.org/Bioethicsforum/Post.aspx?id=5941&blogid=140

Duncombe, J., & Marsden, D. (1996). Whose orgasm is this anyway? Sex work in long-term couple relationships. In J. Weeks & J. Holland (Eds.), *Sexual cultures* (pp. 220–238). Basingstoke, UK: Macmillan. Press.

Dworkin, A. (1987). *Intercourse*. New York, NY: Basic Books.

Ebert, T. (1996). *Ludic feminism and after: Postmodernism, desire, and labor in late capitalism*. Ann Arbor, MI: University of Michigan Press.

Edwards, J. (2010, June 16). Viagra and blindness: Now the FDA is accusing Pfizer of covering up eye problems. *CBS News*. Retrieved from http://www.cbsnews.com/news/viagra-and-blindness-now-the-fda-is-accusing-pfizer-of-covering-up-eye-problems

Ehrenreich, B., & English, D. (1978). *For her own good: 150 years of the experts' advice to women*. Garden City, NJ: Anchor Press/Doubleday.

Elia, J. P. (2003). Queering relationships: Toward a paradigmatic shift. *Journal of Homosexuality, 45*(2-4), 61–86. http://dx.doi.org/10.1300/J082v45n02_03

Elliot, P. (2010). *Debates in transgender, queer, and feminist theory*. Burlington, VT: Ashgate Publishing Ltd.

Ellis, H. (1913). *Studies in the psychology of sex*. Philadelphia, PA: F.A. Davis.

Emerson, J. (1970a). Nothing unusual is happening. In T. Shibutani (Ed.), *Human nature and collective behavior: Essays in honor of Herbert Blumer* (pp. 208–222). Englewood Cliffs, NJ: Prentice Hall.

Emerson, J. (1970b). Behaviour in private places: sustaining definitions of reality in gynaecological examinations. In H. Dreitzel (Ed.), *Recent sociology* (pp. 73–100). New York, NY: Macmillan.

Evans, A., Riley, S., & Shankar, A. (2010). Technologies of sexiness: Theorizing women's engagement in the sexualization of culture. *Feminism & Psychology, 20*(1), 114–131. http://dx.doi.org/10.1177/0959353509351854

Evans, C. B. S. (1931). *Man and woman in marriage*. London, UK: J. Lane.

Fahs, B. (2010). Radical refusals: On the anarchist politics of women choosing asexuality. *Sexualities, 13*(4), 445–461. http://dx.doi.org/10.1177/13634607 10370650

Farrell, J., & Cacchioni, T. (2012). The medicalization of women's sexual pain. *Journal of Sex Research, 49*(4), 328–336. http://dx.doi.org/10.1080/00224499. 2012.688227

Fausto-Sterling, A. (1995). Gender, race, and nation: The comparative anatomy of "Hottentot" women in Europe, 1815–1817. In J. Urla &J. Terry (Eds.), *Deviant bodies: Critical perspectives on difference in science and popular culture* (pp. 19–48). Bloomington, IN: Indiana University Press.

Feldhaus-Dahir, M. (2011). The causes and prevalence of vestibulodynia: A vulvar pain disorder. *Urologic Nursing, 31*, 51–54.

Fishman, J. R. (2004). Manufacturing desire: The commodification of female sexual dysfunction. *Social Studies of Science, 34*(2), 187–218. http://dx.doi.org/10.1177/0306312704043028

Fishman, J., & Mamo, R. (2001). What's in a disorder: A cultural analysis of medical and pharmaceutical constructions of male and female sexual dysfunction. In E. Kaschak & L. Tiefer (Eds.), *A new view of women's sexual problems* (pp. 179–193). Binghampton, NY: Haworth Press.

Foucault, M. (1979). *The history of sexuality* (Vol. 1). London: Allen Lane.

Foucault, M. (1984). Panopticism. In P. Rabinow (Ed.) *The Foucault reader: An introduction to Foucault's thought* (pp. 206–213). London, UK: Penguin.

Frankenberg, R. (1993). *White women: Race matters, the social construction of whiteness.* Minneapolis, MN: University of Minnesota Press.

Friedrich, E. G. (1987). Vulvar vestibulitis syndrome. *Journal of Reproductive Medicine, 32,* 110–114.

Fuss, D. (1991). *Inside/out: Lesbian theories, gay theories.* New York, NY: Routledge.

Gagnon, J. (1977). *Human sexualities.* Glenview, IL: Scott Foresman.

Gavey, N. (1993). Technologies and effects of heterosexual coercion. In S. Wilkinson & C. Kitzinger (Eds.), *Heterosexuality: A feminism & psychology reader* (pp. 93–119). London, UK: Sage Publications.

Gavey, N. (2005). *Just sex? The cultural scaffolding of rape.* London, UK: Routledge.

Gerhard, J. (2000). Revisiting "The myth of the vaginal orgasm": The female orgasm in American sexual thought and second wave feminism. *Feminist Studies, 26,* 449–476. http://dx.doi.org/10.2307/3178545

Ghazizadeh, S., & Nikzad, M. (2004). Botulinum toxin in the treatment of refractory vaginismus. *Obstetrics & Gynecology, 104,* 922–925.

Giddens, A. (1991). *Modernity and self identity.* Oxford, UK: Polity Press.

Giddens, A. (1992). *The transformation of intimacy: Sexuality, love, and eroticism in modern societies.* Cambridge, UK: Polity Press.

Gilfoyle, J., Wilson, J., & Own, B. (1992). Sex, organs, and audiotape: A discourse analytic approach to talking about heterosexual sex and relationships. *Feminism & Psychology, 2*(2), 209–230. http://dx.doi.org/10.1177/095935359222010

Gill, J. T. (1951). *How to hold your husband: A frank psychoanalysis for happy marriage.* Philadelphia: Dorrance.

Glaser, B. G. (2002). Conceptualization: On theory and theorizing using grounded theory. *International Journal of Qualitative Methods, 1,* 23–38.

Glenn, D. R., McVicar, C. M., McClure, N., & Lewis, S. E. (2007). Sildenafil citrate improves sperm motility but causes a premature acrosome reaction in vitro. *Fertility and Sterility, 87*(5), 1064–1070. http://dx.doi.org/10.1016/j.fertnstert.2006.11.017

Goldstein, I. (1997). New field could open up for urologists: Female sexual dysfunction. *Urology Times, 25,* 39.

Goldstein, I., Meston, C. M., Davis, S., & Traish, A. (2006). *Women's sexual function and dysfunction: Study, diagnosis and treatment.* Abingdon, UK: Taylor and Francis Group.

Goodwin, A. J., & Agronin, M. E. (1997). *A woman's guide to overcoming sexual fear and pain*. Oakland, CA: New Harbinger Publications.

Grace, V. M. (2000). Pitfalls of the medical paradigm in chronic pelvic pain. *Best Practice & Research. Clinical Obstetrics & Gynaecology, 14*(3), 525–539. http://dx.doi.org/10.1053/beog.1999.0089

Grace, V. M., & MacBride-Stewart, S. (2007). "How to say it": Women's descriptions of pelvic pain. *Women & Health, 46*(4), 81–98. http://dx.doi.org/10.1300/J013v46n04_05

Graham, C. A., Sanders, S. A., Milhausen, R. R., & McBride, K. R. (2004). Turning on and turning off: A focus group study of the factors that affect women's sexual arousal. *Archives of Sexual Behavior, (33)*6, 527–538.

Graziottin, A., & Brotto, L. A. (2004). Vulvar vestibulitis syndrome: A clinical approach. *Journal of Sex & Marital Therapy, 30*(3), 125–139. http://dx.doi.org/10.1080/00926230490258866

Grogan, K. (2013, June 27th). Sprout resubmits "female Viagra" to FDA. *World News*, Retrieved from http://www.pharmatimes.com/article/13-06-27/Sprout_resubmits_female_Viagra_to_FDA.aspx.

Groneman, C. (1994). Nymphomania: The historical construction of female sexuality. *Signs, 19*(2), 337–367. http://dx.doi.org/10.1086/494887

Gupta, K. (2011). "Screw health": Representations of sex as a health-promoting activity in medical and popular literature. *Journal of Medical Humanities, 32*(2), 127–140. http://dx.doi.org/10.1007/s10912-010-9129-x

Gupta, K., & Cacchioni, T. (2013). Sexual improvement as if your health depends on it: An analysis of contemporary sex manuals. *Feminism & Psychology, 23*(4), 442–458. http://dx.doi.org/10.1177/0959353513498070

Hakim, C. (2010). Erotic capital. *European Sociological Review, 26*(5), 499–518. http://dx.doi.org/10.1093/esr/jcq014

Halberstam, J. J. (1994). F2M: The making of female masculinity. In L. Doan (Ed.), *The lesbian postmodern* (pp. 125–133). New York, NY: Columbia University Press.

Hall, M. (2001). Not tonight dear, I'm deconstructing a headache: Confessions of a lesbian sex therapist. In E. Kaschak & L. Tiefer (Eds.), *A new view of women's sexual problems* (pp. 161–172). Binghamton, NY: Haworth Press.

Halperin, D. M. (Ed.). (1995). *Saint Foucault: Towards a gay hagiography*. New York, NY: Oxford University Press.

Haraway, D. (1999) The virtual speculum in the new world order. In A. Clarke and V. Olesen (Eds.), *Revisioning women, health, and healing* (pp. 49–96). New York, NY: Routledge.

Hartley, H. (2006). The pinking of Viagra culture: Drug industry efforts to create and repackage. *Sexualities, 9*(3), 363–378. http://dx.doi.org/10.1177/1363460706065058

Hartley, H., & Tiefer, L. (2003). Taking a biological turn: The push for a "female Viagra" and the medicalization of women's sexual problems. *Women's Studies Quarterly, 31*, 42–54.

Harvey, L., & Gill, R. (2011). Spicing it up: Sexual entrepreneurs and the sex inspectors. In R. Gill & C. Scharff (Eds.), *New femininities: Postfeminism, neo-liberalism and subjectivity* (pp. 52–67). New York, NY: Palgrave.

Hawkes, G. (1996). *A sociology of sex and sexuality*. Maidenhead, UK: Open University Press.

Hayes, R. D. (2011). Circular and linear modeling of female sexual desire and arousal. *Journal of Sex Research, 48* (2-3), 130–141. doi:10.1080/00224499.2010.548611

Hayes, R., Dennerstein, L., Bennett, C., & Fairley, C. (2008). What is the "true" prevalence of female sexual dysfunctions and does the way we assess these conditions have an impact? *Journal of Sexual Medicine, 5*(4), 777–787. http://dx.doi.org/10.1111/j.1743-6109.2007.00768.x

Heath, C. (1986). *Body movement and speech in medical interaction*. Cambridge, UK: Cambridge University Press. http://dx.doi.org/10.1017/CBO9780511628221

Henslin, J., & Biggs, M. (1971). Dramaturgical desexualisation: The sociology of the vaginal examination. In J. Henslin (Ed.), *Studies in the sociology of sex* (pp. 133–160). New York, NY: Appleton Century Crofts.

Hite, S. (1976). *The Hite report: A nationwide study on female sexuality*. New York, NY: Macmillan.

Hitt, J. (2000, February 20). The second sexual revolution. *New York Times*. Retrieved from http://www.nytimes.com/2000/02/20/magazine/the-second-sexual-revolution.html

Hochschild, A. R. (1983). *The managed heart: The commercialization of human feeling*. Berkeley, CA: University of California Press.

Hodgekiss, A. (2013, May 23). Female Viagra that stimulates the body and the mind could be on the market within three years. *Daily Mail*.

Holland, J., Ramazanoglu, C., Sharpe, S., & Thomson, R. (1998). *The male in the head*. London, UK: Tufnell Press.

Hollway, W. (1984). Women's power in heterosexual sex. *Women's Studies International Forum, 7*(1), 63–68. http://dx.doi.org/10.1016/0277-5395(84)90085-2

Hutton, D. (2003, November). Sex change. *British Vogue*.

Hwancheol, S., Kwanjin, P., Soo-Woong, K., & Jae-Seung, P. (2004). Reasons for discontinuation of sildenafil citrate after successful restoration of erectile function. *Asian Journal of Andrology, 6*, 117–120.

Iasenza, S. (2001). Sex therapy with "a new view." In E. Kaschak & L. Tiefer (Eds.), *A new view of women's sexual problems* (pp. 43–46). Binghamton, NY: Haworth Press.

Irvine, J. (1990). *Disorders of desire: Sex and gender in modern american society.* Philadelphia, PA: Temple University Press.

Jackson, S. (1999). *Heterosexuality in question.* London, UK: Sage Publications.

Jackson, S. (2006). Interchanges: Gender, sexuality and heterosexuality: The complexity (and limits) of heteronormativity. *Feminist Theory, 7*(1), 105–121. http://dx.doi.org/10.1177/1464700106061462

Jackson, S., & Scott, S. (1997). Gut reactions to matters of the heart: Reflections on rationality, irrationality and sexuality. *Sociological Review, 45*(4), 551–575. http://dx.doi.org/10.1111/1467-954X.00077

Jackson, S., & Scott, S. (2001). Embodying orgasm: Gendered power relations and sexual pleasure. In E. Kaschak & L. Tiefer (Eds.), *A new view of women's sexual problems* (pp. 99–110). Binghamton, NY: Haworth Press.

Jannini, E., Lombardo, F., Salacone, P., Gandini, L., & Lenzi, A. (2004). Treatment of sexual dysfunctions secondary to male infertility with sildenafil citrate. *Fertility and Sterility, 81*(3), 705–707.

Jeffreys, S. (1990). *Anti-climax: A feminist critique of the sexual revolution.* London, UK: Women's Press.

Jeffreys, S. (1997). *The spinster and her enemies: Feminism and sexuality, 1880–1930.* Melbourne: Spinifex Press.

Jetter, A. (2010, February). Lust caution. *Vogue,* 206–209.

Johnson, M. L. (Ed.). (2002). *Jane sexes it up: True confessions of feminist desire.* New York, NY: Four Walls Eight Windows.

Jones, C. & Porter, R. (Eds.). (1997). *Reassessing Foucault: Power, medicine, and the body.* New York, NY: Routledge.

Kaler, A. (2006). Unreal women: Sex, gender, identity and the lived experience of vulvar pain. *Feminist Review, 82*(1), 50–75. http://dx.doi.org/10.1057/palgrave.fr.9400262

Kaplan, H. S. (1977). Hypoactive sexual desire. *Journal of Sex & Marital Therapy, 3*(1), 3–9. doi I:10.1080/00926237708405343

Kapsalis, T. (1997). *Public privates: Performing gynecology from both ends of the speculum.* Durham, NC: Duke University Press.

Kaschak, E. & Tiefer, L. (Eds.). (2001). *A new view of women's sexual problems.* Binghamptom, NY: Haworth Press.

Katz, S., & Marshall, B. (2003). New sex for old: Lifestyle, consumerism, and the ethics of aging well. *Journal of Aging Studies, 17*(1), 3–16. http://dx.doi.org/10.1016/S0890-4065(02)00086-5

Katz, D., & Tabisel, R. (2002). *Private pain: It's about life not just sex.* Plainview, NY: Katz-Tabi Publications.

Kimmel, A. J. (1988). *Ethics and values in applied social research.* Newbury Park, CA: Sage.

King, S. (2006). *Pink ribbons, inc.: Breast cancer and the politics of philanthropy.* Minneapolis, MN: University of Minnesota Press.

King, S. (2010). Pink ribbons inc.: The emergence of cause-related marketing and the corporatization of the breast cancer movement. In P. Saukko (Ed.), *Governing the female body gender, health, and networks of power* (pp. 85–111). Albany, NY: State University of New York Press.

Kinsey, A. C., Pomeroy, W. B., & Martin, C. E. (1948). *Sexual behaviour in the human male.* Philadelphia, PA: W.B. Saunders.

Kipnis, L. (2006). *Bound and gagged pornography and the politics of fantasy in America.* Durham, NC: Duke University Press.

Kleinplatz, P. J. (Ed.). (2012). *New directions in sex therapy: Innovations and alternatives* (2nd ed.). New York, NY: Routledge.

Klotz, T., Mathers, M., Klotz, R., & Sommer, F. (2005). Why do patients with erectile dysfunction abandon effective therapy with Sildenafil (Viagra)? *International Journal of Impotence Research, 17*(1), 2–4. http://dx.doi.org/10.1038/sj.ijir.3901252

Koedt, A. (1973). The myth of the vaginal orgasm. In A. Koedt, E. Levine, & A. Rapone (Eds.), *Radical feminism* (pp. 198–207). New York, NY: Quadrangle Books.

Koch, P. B., Mansfield, P. K., Thurau, D., & Carey, M. (2005). "Feeling frumpy": The relationships between body image and sexual response changes in midlife women. *Journal of Sex Research, 42*(3), 215–223. http://dx.doi.org/10.1080/00224490509552276

Kong, D. (1999, October 22). Doubts heard over sexual dysfunction gathering. *Boston Globe,* B1, B6.

Krane, R. J., Siroky, M. B., & Goldstein, I. (Eds.). (1983). *Male sexual dysfunction.* Boston, MA: Little, Brown.

Krychman, M. L., & Kingsberg, S. A. (2013). Female sexual disorders: Treatment options in the pipeline. *Formulary, 48,* 113.

Labuski, C. (2013). Deferred desire: The asexuality of chronic genital pain. In K.J. Cerankowski & M. Milks (Eds.), *The asexuality anthology* (pp. 302–325). New York, NY: Routledge.

Landau, E. (2013, June 5). Sex is doctor's life's work. *CNN health.* Retrieved from http://www.cnn.com/2013/05/31/health/lifeswork-sex-medicine

Landry, T., Bergeron, S., Dupuis, M., & Desrochers, G. (2008). The treatment of. provoked Vestibulodynia: A critical review. *Clinical Journal of Pain, 24*(2), 155–171. http://dx.doi.org/10.1097/AJP.0b013e31815aac4d

Laumann, E. O., Gagnon, J. M., & Michaels, S. (1994). *The social organization of sexuality: Sexual practices in the United States.* Chicago, IL: University of Chicago Press.

Laumann, E. O., Paik, A., & Rosen, S. C. (1999). Sexual dysfunction in the United States: Prevalence and predictors. *Journal of the American Medical Association, 281*(6), 537–544. http://dx.doi.org/10.1001/jama.281.6.537

Lavie, M., & Willig, C. (2005). I don't feel like melting butter: An interpretative phenomenological analysis of the experience of "inorgasmia". *Psychology & Health, 20*(1), 115–128. http://dx.doi.org/10.1080/08870440412331 296044

Lavie-Ajayi, M., & Joffe, H. (2009). Social representations of female orgasm. *Journal of Health Psychology, 14*(1), 98–107. http://dx.doi.org/10.1177/1359 105308097950

Leman, K. (2003). *Sheet music: Uncovering the secrets of sexual intimacy in marriage.* Carol Stream, IL: Tyndale House Publishers.

Light, D. (2000). The sociological character of health-care markets. In G.L. Albrecht, R. Fitzpatrick, & S. Scrimshaw (Eds.), *Handbook of social studies in health and medicine* (pp. 394–408). London, UK: Sage Publications.

Liswood, R., & Davis, B. (1961). *A marriage doctor speaks her mind about sex.* New York, NY: Ace Books.

Loe, M. (2001). Fixing broken masculinity: Viagra as a technology for the production of gender and sexuality. *Sexuality and Culture, 5*(3), 97–125. doi 10.1007/s12119-001-1032-1

Loe, M. (2004a). *The rise of Viagra: How the little blue pill changed sex in America.* New York, NY: New York University Press.

Loe, M. (2004b). Sex and the senior woman: Pleasure and danger in the viagra era. *Sexualities, 7*(3), 303–326. http://dx.doi.org/10.1177/136346070 4044803

Lundberg, F., & Farnham, M. F. (1947). *Modern woman: The lost sex.* New York, NY: Harper & Brothers.

Marcuse, H. (1955). *Eros and civilization.* London, UK: Routledge.

Marriott, C., & Thompson, A. R. (2008). Managing threats to femininity: Personal and interpersonal experience of living with vulvar pain. *Psychology & Health, 23*(2), 243–258. http://dx.doi.org/10.1080/14768320601168185

Marshall, B.L. (2012). Medicalization and the refashioning of age-related limits on sexuality. *Journal of Sex Research, 49*(4), 337–343. http://dx.doi.org/ 10.1080/00224499.2011.644597

Martin, E. (1994). *Flexible bodies: Tracking immunity in American culture from the days of polio to the age of AIDS.* Boston: Beacon Press.

Masters, W. H., & Johnson, V. E. (1966). *Human sexual response.* Boston, MA: Little Brown.

Masters, W. H., Johnson, V. E., & Kolodny, R. C. (1986). *Masters and Johnson on sex and human loving.* Boston: Little, Brown.

McCaughey, M., & French, C. (2001). Women's sex-toy parties: Technology, orgasm, and commodification. *Sexuality & Culture*, 5(3), 77–96. http://dx.doi.org/10.1007/s12119-001-1031-2

McKay, M. (1989). Vulvodynia: A multifactorial clinical problem. *Archives of Dermatology*, 125(2), 256–262. http://dx.doi.org/10.1001/archderm.1989.01670140108021

McNay, L. (1992). *Feminism and Foucault*. Oxford, UK: Polity.

McRobbie, A. (2006) Four technologies of young womanhood, paper presented at TU-Berlin Zentrum für Interdisziplinare Frauen und Geschlecterforschung, October 31.

Meana, M. (2010). Elucidating women's (hetero) sexual desire: Definitional challenges and content expansion. *Journal of Sex Research*, 47(2-3), 104–122. http://dx.doi.org/10.1080/00224490903402546

Metzl, J., & Kirkland, A. R. (Eds). (2010). *Against health: How health became the new morality*. New York, NY: New York University Press.

Mitka, M. (2000). Some men who take Viagra die – why? *Journal of the American Medical Association*, 283, 590–593.

Morgensen, S. L. (2011). The biopolitics of settler colonialism: Right here, right now. *Settler Colonial Studies*, 1(1), 52–76. http://dx.doi.org/10.1080/2201473X.2011.10648801

Moynihan, R. (2003). The making of a disease: Female sexual dysfunction. *British Medical Journal*, 326(7379), 45–47. http://dx.doi.org/10.1136/bmj.326.7379.45

Moynihan, R., & Mintzes, B. (2010). *Sex, lies and pharmaceuticals: How drug companies plan to profit from female sexual dysfunction*. Vancouver, BC: Greystone Books.

Neuhaus, J. (2000). The importance of being orgasmic: Sexuality, gender, and marital sex manuals in the United States. *Journal of the History of Sexuality*, 9, 447–473.

Nicholls, L. (2008). Putting the New View classification scheme to an empirical test. *Feminism & Psychology*, 18(4), 515–526. http://dx.doi.org/10.1177/0959353508096180

Nicolson, P. (1993). Deconstructing sexology: Understanding the pathologization of female sexuality. *Journal of Reproductive and Infant Psychology*, 11(4), 191–201. http://dx.doi.org/10.1080/02646839308403218

Nicolson, P., & Burr, J. (2003). What is "normal" about women's (hetero) sexual desire and orgasm? A report of an in-depth interview. *Social Science & Medicine*, 57(9), 1735–1745. http://dx.doi.org/10.1016/S0277-9536(03)00012-1

Nurius, P. S. (1983). Mental health implications of sexual orientation. *Journal of Sex Research*, 19(2), 119–136. http://dx.doi.org/10.1080/00224498309551174

Oakley, A. (2005). *The Ann Oakley reader: Gender, women and social science*. Bristol, UK: Policy Press.

O'Connell Davidson, J., & Layder, D. (1994). *Methods, sex, and madness*. New York, NY: Routledge. http://dx.doi.org/10.4324/9780203423455

O'Connor, A. M. (2005, October 2). Dr. Berman's sex Rx. *Los Angeles Times*. Retrieved from http://articles.latimes.com/print/2005/oct/02/magazine/tm-sexresearch40

Ogden, G. (2001). The taming of the screw: Reflections on "a new view of women's sexual problems". In E. Kaschak & L. Tiefer (Eds.), *A new view of women's sexual problems* (pp. 17–22). Binghampton, NY: Haworth Press.

O'Rourke, M. (2005). On the eve of a queer-straight future: Notes toward an antinormative heteroerotic. *Feminism & Psychology*, 15(1), 111–116. http://dx.doi.org/10.1177/0959353505049713

Pacik, P. T. (2009). Botox treatment for vaginismus. *Plastic and Reconstructive Surgery*, 124(6), 455e–456e. http://dx.doi.org/10.1097/PRS.0b013e3181bf7f11

Pacik, P. T. (2011). Vaginismus: Review of current concepts and treatment using botox injections, bupivacaine injections, and progressive dilation with the patient under anesthesia. *Aesthetic Plastic Surgery*, 35(6), 1160–1164. http://dx.doi.org/10.1007/s00266-011-9737-5

Pacik, P. T., & Cole, J. B. (2010). *When sex seems impossible: Stories of vaginismus and how you can achieve intimacy*. Manchester, UK: Odyne Publishing.

Palmer, E. (2013). Pfizer's Viagra patent in Europe expires today: As many as 20 generic drugmakers expected to flood the market in U.K, Europe. Available online at http://www.fiercepharma.com/story/pfizers-viagra-patent-europe-expires-today/2013-06-21; accessed 18 December 2013.

Paulus, W., Strehler, E., Zhang, M., Jelinkova, L., El-Danasouri, I., & Sterzik, K. (2002). Benefit of vaginal sildenafil citrate in assisted reproduction therapy. *Fertility and Sterility*, 77(4), 846–847. http://dx.doi.org/10.1016/S0015-0282(01)03272-1

Payne, K.A., Bergeron, S., Khalifé, S., & Binik, Y.M. (2006). Assessment, treatment strategies and outcome results: Perspective of pain specialists. In I. Goldstein, C. M., Meston, S. Davis, & A. Traish (Eds.), *Women's sexual function and dysfunction: Study, diagnosis, and treatment* (pp. 471–479). New York, NY: Taylor & Francis.

Peer Commentaries. (2005). Peer commentaries on Binik's "Should dyspareunia be retained as a sexual dysfunction in DSM-V? A painful classification decision". *Archives of Sexual Behavior*, 34, 23–61.

Perkins, J. (2011, February). Sex, drugs, and the quest for the female Viagra. *San Diego Magazine*, 32, 34.

Petersen, A., & Bunton, R. (Eds.). (2000). *Foucault, health and medicine*. New York, NY: Routledge.

Plummer, K. (2007). Queers, bodies, and postmodern sexualities: A note on revisiting the sexual in symbolic interactionism. In M. Kimmel (Ed.), *The sexual self* (pp. 16–30). Nashville, TN: Vanderbilt University Press.

Polzer, J. C., & Knabe, S. M. (2012). From desire to disease: Human papillomavirus (HPV) and the medicalization of nascent female sexuality. *Journal of Sex Research, 49*(4), 344–352.

Popenoe, P. (1925). *Modern marriage: A handbook*. New York, NY: Macmillan.

Portman, D. J., Bachmann, G. A., & Simon, J.A. (2013). Ospemifene, a novel selective estrogen receptor modulator for treating dyspareunia associated with postmenopausal vulvar and vaginal atrophy. *Menopause, 20*, 623–630.

Potts, A. (2002). *The science/fiction of sex: Feminist deconstruction of the vocabularies of heterosex*. New York, NY: Routledge.

Potts, A., Gavey, N., Grace, V. M., & Vares, T. (2003). The downside of Viagra: Women's experiences and concerns. *Sociology of Health & Illness, 25*(7), 697–719. http://dx.doi.org/10.1046/j.1467-9566.2003.00366.x

Potts, A., & Tiefer, L. (2006). Introduction. *Sexualities, 9*(3), 267–272. http://dx.doi.org/10.1177/1363460706065048

Prause, N., & Graham, C. A. (2007). Asexuality: Classification and characterization. *Archives of Sexual Behavior, 36*(3), 341–356. http://dx.doi.org/10.1007/s10508-006-9142-3

Przybylo, E. (2011). Crisis and safety: The asexual in sexusociety. *Sexualities, 14*(4), 444–461. http://dx.doi.org/10.1177/1363460711406461

Przybylo, E. (2013). Producing facts: Empirical asexuality and the scientific study of sex. *Feminism & Psychology, 23*(2), 224–242. http://dx.doi.org/10.1177/0959353512443668

Razack, S. (2000). Gendered racial violence and spatialized justice: The murder of Pamela George. *Canadian Journal of Law and Society, 15*(2), 91–130. http://dx.doi.org/10.1017/S0829320100006384

Renold, E., & Ringrose, J. (2008). Regulation and rupture: Mapping tween and teenage girls' resistance to the heterosexual matrix. *Feminist Theory, 9*(3), 313–338. http://dx.doi.org/10.1177/1464700108095854

Rich, A. (1980). Compulsory heterosexuality and lesbian existence. *Signs, 5*(4), 631–660. http://dx.doi.org/10.1086/493756

Richardson, D. (Ed.). (1996). *Theorizing heterosexuality: Telling it straight*. Maidenhead, UK: Open University Press.

Riessman, C. K. (1983). Women and medicalization: a new perspective. *Social Policy, 14*, 3–18.

Roberts, C., Kippax, S., Waldby, C., & Crawford, J. (1995). Faking it. *Women's Studies International Forum, 18*, 523–532.

Robinson, I., Ziss, K., Ganza, B., Katz, S., & Robinson, E. (1991). Twenty years of the sexual revolution 1965–1985. An update. *Journal of Marriage and the Family, 53*(1), 216–220. http://dx.doi.org/10.2307/353145

Rochon Ford, A. & Saibil, D. (Eds.). (2009). *The push to prescribe*. Toronto, ON: Women's Press.

Rose, N.S. (2007). *Politics of life itself: Biomedicine, power, and subjectivity in the twenty-first century*. Princeton, NJ: Princeton University Press.

Rose, N., & Novas, C. (2005). Biological citizenship. In A. Ong & S.J. Collier (Eds.), *Global assemblages: Technology, politics, and ethics as anthropological problems* (pp. 439–463). Malden, MA: Blackwell.

Rubin, G. (1984). Thinking sex: Notes for a radical theory of the politics of sexuality. In C.S. Vance (Ed.), *Pleasure and danger: Exploring female sexuality* (pp. 267–319). Boston, MA: Routledge & Kegan Paul.

Salamone, G. (2008, March 25). Viagra reaches the 10-year milestone. *Daily News America*. Retrieved from http://www.nydailynews.com/life-style/health/viagra-reaches-10-year-milestone-article-1.291510

Scherrer, K. S. (2008). Coming to an asexual identity: Negotiating identity, negotiating desire. *Sexualities, 11*(5), 621–641. http://dx.doi.org/10.1177/1363460708094269

Schlichter, A. (2004). Queer at last? Straight intellectuals and the desire for transgression. *GLQ: A Journal of Lesbian and Gay Studies, 10*, 543–564.

Seal, B. N., Bradford, A., & Meston, C. M. (2009). The association between body esteem and sexual desire among college women. *Archives of Sexual Behavior, 38*(5), 866–872.

Shafik, A., & Eli-Sibai, O. (2000). Vaginismus: Results of the treatment with botulin toxin. *Journal of Gynecology, 20*(3), 300–302. http://dx.doi.org/10.1080/01443610050009674

Shaw, I. (2002). How lay are lay beliefs? *Health, 6*(3), 287–299. http://dx.doi.org/10.1177/136345930200600302

Sher, G., & Fisch, J. D. (2000). Vaginal sildenafil (Viagra): A preliminary report of a novel method to improve uterine artery blood flow and endometrial development in patients undergoing IVF. *Human Reproduction, 78*(5), 1073–1076.

Simon, W. (1996). *Postmodern sexualities*. London, UK: Routledge.

Skeggs, B. (1997). *Formations of class & gender: Becoming respectable*. New York, NY: Sage.

Smart, C. (1996). Desperately seeking post-heterosexual women. In J. Holland & L. Adkins (Eds.), *Sex, sensibility, and the gendered body* (pp. 222–241). New York, NY: St. Martin's Press.

Smith-Rosenberg, C. (1975). The female world of love and ritual: Relations between women in nineteenth-century America. *Signs, 1*(1), 1–29.

Stein, A. (2009). *Heal pelvic pain*. New York, NY: McGraw-Hill.

Storms, M. (1979). Sexual orientation and self-perception. In P. Pliner, K. R. Blankstein, & I. M. Spiegel (Eds.), *Perception of emotion in self and others* (pp. 165–180). New York, NY: Plenum.

Strong, P. (1979). Sociological imperialism and the profession of medicine: a critical examination of the thesis of medical imperialism. *Social Science and Medicine 13A* (2), 199–215.

Thomas, C. (Ed.). (2000). Straight with a twist: Queer theory and the subject of heterosexuality. Urbana, IL: University of Illinois Press.

Thompson, S. (1990). Putting a big thing into a little hole: Teenage girls' accounts of sexual initiation. *Journal of Sex Research, 27*(3), 341–361. http://dx.doi.org/10.1080/00224499009551564

Thompson, S. (1995). *Going all the way: Teenage girls' tales of sex, romance, and pregnancy*. New York, NY: Hill and Wang.

Tiefer, L. (1983). Sexual excitement/sexual peace: The place of masturbation in adult relationships. *Psychology of Women Quarterly, 8*(1), 107–109. http://dx.doi.org/10.1177/036168438300800102

Tiefer, L. (1986). In pursuit of the perfect penis: The medicalization of male sexuality. *American Behavioral Scientist, 29*(5), 579–599. http://dx.doi.org/10.1177/000276486029005006

Tiefer, L. (1995). *Sex is not a natural act and other essays*. Boulder, CO: Westview Press.

Tiefer, L. (1999, October). "Female sexual dysfunction" alert: A new disorder invented for women. *Sojourner: The Women's Forum*, 11.

Tiefer, L. (2001). Arriving at a "new view" of women's sexual problems: Background, theory, and activism. In E. Kaschak & L. Tiefer (Eds.), *A new view of women's sexual problems* (pp. 63–98). Binghamton, NY: Haworth Press.

Tiefer, L. (2002). Arriving at a "new view" of women's sexual problems: Background, theory, and activism. *Women & Therapy, 24*(1-2), 63–98. http://dx.doi.org/10.1300/J015v24n01_12

Tiefer, L. (2005). Dyspareunia is the only valid sexual dysfunction and certainly the only important one. *Archives of Sexual Behavior, 34*(1), 49–51. http://dx.doi.org/10.1007/s10508-005-7477-8

Tiefer, L. (2006a). Sex therapy as a humanistic enterprise. *Sexual and Relationship Therapy, 21*(3), 359–375. http://dx.doi.org/10.1080/14681990600740723

Tiefer, L. (2006b). The Viagra phenomenon. *Sexualities, 9*(3), 273–294. http://dx.doi.org/10.1177/1363460706065049

Tiefer, L. (2007). Beneath the veneer: The troubled past and future of sexual medicine. *Journal of Sex & Marital Therapy, 33*(5), 473–477. http://dx.doi.org/10.1080/00926230701480521

Tiefer, L. (2008). The new view in activism and academics 10 years on. *Feminism & Psychology*, *18*(4), 451–456. http://dx.doi.org/10.1177/09593535080 95527

Tiefer, L. (2012). Medicalizations and demedicalizations of sexuality therapies. *Journal of Sex Research*, *49*(4), 311–318. http://dx.doi.org/10.1080/00224499. 2012.678948

Tiefer, L., & Tavris, C. (1999). Viagra for women is the wrong Rx. *Los Angeles Times*, B9.

Tiefer, L., Witczak, K., & Heath, I. (2013). A call to challenge the "selling of sickness". *British Medical Journal*, *13*, 346.

Tolman, D. L. (2001). Female adolescent sexuality: An argument for a developmental perspective on the new view of women's sexual problems. In E. Kaschak & L. Tiefer (Eds.), *A new view of women's sexual problems* (pp. 195–210). Binghamton, NY: Haworth Press.

Twigg, J., Cohen, R., Nettleton, S., & Wolkowitz, C. (2011). Special issue on body work in health and social care. *Sociology of Health & Illness*, *33*, 266–279.

Tyler, M. (2004). Managing between the sheets: Lifestyle magazines and the management of sexuality in everyday life. *Sexualities*, *7*(1), 81–106. http://dx.doi.org/10.1177/1363460704040144

United States (2000). Food and Drug Administration. 2000 Draft guidance for industry female sexual dysfunction: Clinical development of drug products for treatment. Washington, DC. Available at http://www.fda.gov/Science Research/SpecialTopics/WomensHealthResearch/ucm133202.htm.

United States (2010). Food and Drug Administration. Transcript for the June 18, 2010, meeting of the Advisory Committee for Reproductive Health Drugs. Washington, DC. Available at http://www.fda.gov/downloads/ AdvisoryCommittees/CommitteesMeetingMaterials/Drugs/Reproductive HealthDrugsAdvisoryCommittee/UCM248753.pdf.

Vance, C. (1984). *Pleasure & danger: Exploring female sexuality*. Boston, MA: Routledge.

Van de Velde, T. H. (1930). *Ideal marriage; its physiology and technique*. Trans. S. Browne. New York, NY: Random House.

Viagra patent tossed out by the Supreme Court (2012, November 8). *CBC News*. Retrieved from http://www.cbc.ca/news/business/viagra-patent-tossed-out-by-supreme-court-1.1216466

Voss, B. (2015, January 21). Vagina Monologues playwright responds after show cancelled for not being trans inclusive. *Advocate.com*.

Wayman, C.P., Baxter, D., Turner, L., Van Der Graaf, P.H., & Naylor, A.M. (2010). UK-414, 495, a selective inhibitor of neutral endopeptidase, potentiates pelvic nerve stimulated increases in female genital blood flow in the anaesthetized rabbit. *British Journal of Pharmacology, 160*(1), 51–59. http://dx.doi.org/10.1111/j.1476-5381.2010.00691.x

Weedon, C. (1987). *Feminist practice and postructuralist theory.* Oxford, UK: Blackwell Press.

Weeks, J. (1991). *Against nature: Essays on history, sexuality and identity.* London, UK: Rivers Oram Press.

Williams, S. J. (2001). Sociological imperialism and the profession of medicine revisited: Where are we now? *Sociology of Health & Illness, 23*(2), 135–158. http://dx.doi.org/10.1111/1467-9566.00245

Wilson, D. (2010, June 17). Push to market pill stirs debate on sexual desire. *New York Times.* Retrieved from http://www.nytimes.com/2010/06/17/business/17sexpill.html?_r=1&

Wood, L. F., & Dickinson, R. L. (1939). *Harmony in marriage.* New York, NY: Round Table Press.

Working Group for a New View of Women's Sexual Problems. (2001). A new view of women's sexual problems. In E. Kaschak and L. Tiefer (Eds.), *A new view of women's sexual problems* (pp. 1–8). Binghampton, NY: Haworth Press.

Zola, I. K. (1983). *Socio-medical inquiries.* Philadelphia, PA: Temple University Press.

# Index

Milton Keynes UK
Ingram Content Group UK Ltd.
UKHW012227190424
441406UK00001B/112